Private Lives in Public Places

DIANNE WILLCOCKS, SHEILA PEACE,
and LEONIE KELLAHER

Private Lives in Public Places

A research-based critique of residential life in local
authority old people's homes

with a foreword by
M. Powell Lawton

Tavistock Publications
London and New York

First published in 1987 by
Tavistock Publications Ltd
11 New Fetter Lane, London EC4P 4EE

Published in the USA by
Tavistock Publications
in association with Methuen, Inc.
29 West 35th Street, New York, NY 10001

Typeset by Mayhew Typesetting, Bristol
Printed and bound in Great Britain
at the University Press, Cambridge

British Library Cataloguing in Publication Data
Willcocks, Dianne M.
    Private lives in public places: a research-based
    critique of residential life in local authority old
    people's homes.
    1. Old age homes — Great Britain
    I. Title   II. Peace, Sheila M.   III. Kellaher,
    Leonie A.
    362.6'1'0941   HV1481.G52
    ISBN 0-422-79150-4
    ISBN 0-422-79160-1 Pbk

Library of Congress Cataloging in Publication Data
Willcocks, Dianne M.
    Private lives in public places.
    (Social Science Paperbacks:)
    Bibliography: p.
    Includes index.
    1. Old age homes — Great Britain. 2. Aged —
Institutional care — Great Britain. I. Peace, Sheila M.
II. Kellaher, Leonie A.   III. Title.   IV. Series.
HV 1454.2.G7W55   1987   362.1'6'0941   86-14485
ISBN 0-422-79150-4
ISBN 0-422-79160-1 (pbk.)

Contents

Acknowledgements

In researching this book, we encroached considerably upon the home-ground of the many old people in the hundred establishments. We would like to thank them first of all for making us welcome and allowing us to learn so much about their special way of life in residential care. We hope this book represents their views fittingly, and to their benefit. Amongst the homes in the wider study we would single out for special thanks the three homes in which we undertook our detailed work, and also the residents and staff in the eight homes which participated in our pilot work and in group discussions. To all the staff in all the homes we are indebted. They gave their time to talk to us, formally in interviews and also less formally. They were open and generous with information when it was not always easy for them to reconcile their own criticisms of practice with the need to carry on despite difficult and sometimes stressful situations. There are many other people in the local authorities we would like to thank: the planners and architects who took part in the detailed studies and provided a most valuable context for our understanding of residential processes; and for allowing us access to a sample of homes in their authorities we must thank the Directors of Social Services in the twenty-nine local authorities in which the hundred homes were located.

The project was funded by the Works Division of the Department of Health and Social Security. They were encouraging throughout as well as being most receptive of our attempts to integrate the social facets of residential living with the physical or built element which most concerned them. Particularly, we must thank Mick Kemp and Elizabeth Young from Works Division; Hazel Canter and Peter Lawrence from Policy Division.

Setting up the survey with residents and staff in the homes was an enormous task. We were supported in this by John O'Brien and Nick Moon at National Opinion Polls. The sampling was also undertaken by NOP and to Chris Russell-Vick who produced the sampling report we are also indebted. Many colleagues at the Polytechnic of North London have been involved in the evolution of this study from its inception right through to this book. We particularly acknowledge the work of Sue O'Brien who was project assistant throughout. Farida Beverley undertook a comprehensive literature search in the preliminary stages and Jane Cook gave technical assistance in the designing of question-naires. Robin Kellaher validated the visual game at pilot stage. Once the main study was underway, a number of people assisted with data collection. A sensitive and dedicated body of interviewers was recruited and trained by NOP and we would like to thank them. Additionally, the following colleagues were involved in the collection of special data sets: Geoff Hunt, David Kitson, and Clive Wood who visited many of the homes to appraise the physical facilities.

At various stages we have made demands upon our colleagues for computing support. At the early stages of analysis Jim Ring and Shai Faruqui gave valuable and patient assistance in handling a large and complicated data set. We could not have achieved anything without their imaginative and sustained help. At the later stage of secondary analysis, we continued to make demands upon the ingenuity of colleagues with computing expertise. They never failed to meet the intellectual challenges with which we faced them, and we are most grateful to Ian James and to Dave Phillips. The secondary analysis of the data was funded by a grant from the Economic and Social Research Council. The shape that this book has taken is due in considerable part to the insights and elaborations of the data which the ESRC grant allowed us to achieve, and we would like to thank them for supporting us in this.

We have received secretarial support from many staff in the Department of Applied Social Studies and want to mention particularly Pat Howe, Pat Flavell, and Maureen Fedarb. Others who have helped have been Caroline Nonweiler, Margaret Leaver, and Steve Buzzard. Finally, Carol Cox undertook illustrations and graphics for us. To all these people we are indebted, and here we must not forget to acknowledge John Hall who was involved in the project from the start and brought to bear his skills in dealing with budgets and financing.

The Polytechnic of North London supported the project by giving space and scarce facilities, and the Faculty of Social Studies has sustained an interest throughout and supported us in establishing CESSA (Centre for Environmental and Social Studies in Ageing) within the Faculty in 1983. Our CESSA advisory group has given us invaluable guidance since then and we would like to thank them all. Finally, our colleagues in gerontology have always been encouraging and have given us an invaluable perspective on the development of our ideas.

This report is based on research funded by the Department of Health and Social Security. The views expressed are those of the authors and not necessarily those of the DHSS or of any other Government Department.

Foreword

M. Powell Lawton

This new analysis of a genre of residential care follows in a tradition of brilliant studies, including the classic study by Peter Townsend which focused on social deprivation in homes for the aged, and those of the architect Alan Lipman, which have elevated the physical features of the residence into their rightful place as a salient component of the context of care. The authors perceive clearly the continuing evolution of the home for the aged in the late twentieth century and begin their scrutiny not only with a social and physical, but also with a clearly political orientation. This enlargement of the nature of the problem is at one and the same time an excitingly original feature and one that is certain to arouse controversy.

If this author may be permitted an oversimplification as a way of beginning this introduction, Mss Willcocks, Peace, and Kellaher suggest that the problems of residential care for the elderly begin with a burden inherited from past history: a tradition of social control by example, whereby impoverished institutional inmates pay the price for their dependence by relinquishing property, social rights, and ultimately self.

This ideological basis and its contemporary manifestations are carefully traced, both through empirical data from a major study of British homes, and through an incisive stripping away of some of the pretences associated with the manicured 'for-publication' version of care as delivered today. They argue persuasively that the 'home' is anything but a domicile. The right to privacy, to self-chosen presentation of the best in the self, to knowledgeable risk-taking, and to some presence in the larger community, are seen as difficult to achieve in the institution. Despite a commitment to altruism and resident self-determination, staff are swept into the pursuit of organizational, rather than residents', goals.

How can those who perceive these deficiencies in the present system move beyond the status quo? Interestingly, the authors do not take the easy solution of recommending the end of the home for the aged. The replacement model is less a place than an embodiment of principles, of which the 'normalization' concept is central. This final statement no doubt will be widely quoted and also will constitute a taking-off point for alternative suggestions.

Viewing the ways that the many variants of residential care have evolved in all industrialized societies, one can see how universal these criticisms are. Whether one has in mind an English geriatric hospital, an American nursing home, warden housing, or congregate housing (*logement-foyers*), it is clear that mortification of the individual occurs pervasively in the name of goals such as safety, tender loving care, cleanliness, and efficiency. Although this book treats only one of these many environmental types, the English home for the aged, the classes of intrusion into personal autonomy are universal, a matter of degree rather than specificity.

The science of gerontology is advanced considerably by the authors' extremely readable theoretical orientation, which argues strongly for the importance of place and its meaning among all that comprises the person's life. Drawing upon the richest concepts in this area, they add their own conception of environment to the socio-political analysis of homes for the aged. Especially noteworthy is their careful avoidance of the idea that the structure, decor, or furniture arrangements in these environments exert a causal influence on the behaviour of passive organisms. They reject environmental determinism. They develop at length the idea that physical environment is only one component of a larger whole, one that is shaped by ideology as well as professional caregivers. Under some conditions, the way homes for the aged are designed may inhibit or facilitate certain behaviours. Their analysis of how thoughtful design can make more probable the resident's achievement of personal goals is thought-provoking and directly useful to the designer.

Another welcome analysis of a neglected topic deals with the people who staff homes for the aged. Their day-to-day transactions with residents are seen to be a function not only of the caregiving tasks, but also of their personal backgrounds and the social ideology of the larger society. No wonder staff feel conflict in attempting to meet goals that flow variously from their personal needs, residents' needs, the organization's needs, and the social polity's needs. A host of approaches to staff training and supervision are suggested by the data and the discussion.

The characteristics of the residents are, of course, all-important in defining what care ought to be given. The failings of the institution may even have differential significance for different residents, an influence that augments or moderates the overall negativity of external control, impersonality, and levelling of individuality. It is of interest to note that the residents of these homes shared some characteristics with those in American nursing homes. The socially unconnected person is overrepresented – the never-married or widowed, for example. This imbalance suggests that the social deprivation may itself be a reason for some people's entering the institution, perhaps in the absence of the usual reasons for admission such as physical or mental impairment. Such an excess risk for the unafflicted suggests, first, that some of the wrong people are going to homes for the aged and, second, that the cluster of institutional negatives may have a particularly deleterious effect on the independent strivings of those who are too competent for the over-provident environment.

What about those whose competence, in mental and physical terms, lies on the other side of the distribution? This is a question needing in-depth research of the type these authors have applied to the somewhat healthier population who live in homes for the aged. For example, does having decision-making power in risky situations have the same meaning for the minorities who were bedridden, memory-impaired, or disoriented? In the United States close to three-quarters of nursing home residents fall into this highly-impaired group. It would seem that the balance and dynamic transactions between personal needs and the socio-physical care environment require continued study in order to know how much control, how much autonomy, or how much personal space are potentially usable by people with different levels of illness or disability. A second such research need is for a longitudinal look at how personal control functions or is desired as the person's health changes.

In conclusion, it is easy to agree with the authors' conclusions, that there is no existing institution, or target group of residential clients, whose purposes would not be better served by a turn toward normalization, an emphasis on social rather than physical care, and deliberate attempts to augment opportunities for the exercise of autonomy.

M. Powell Lawton, Ph.D.
Director of Behavioral Research
Philadelphia Geriatric Center
Philadelphia, Pennsylvania, USA
June, 1986

CHAPTER 1

The concept of home

'Private lives in public places'. With this title we catch our first glimpse of what appear to be conflicting interests in public provision of residential care for elderly people. A consideration of a number of opposing forces within residential caring forms the central theme of this book, which contrasts the rhetoric of policy with observed practice. Taking an historical perspective, we can trace the origins of residential provision from the Victorian workhouse to the purpose built, forty-bedded home typical of public provision today. In so doing we can see an increasing emphasis being placed on normality, client self-determination, and community integration.

Without doubt, these are commendable and worthwhile goals to pursue, yet attempts to implement them often generate a series of contradictions. For example, the study upon which this text hinges reveals that local authorities often voice an ideal philosophy of care as one in which residents retain control of their private world yet at the same time receive care and protection. But the experiential reality for old people may be far removed from this ideal balance, and residential life can become something of a battleground between individual and organizational needs. A related contradiction is seen in the statement of intent that residential establishments should be modelled upon domestic rather than institutional ideas. In reality, the ideal of providing a 'homely' setting is a genteel facade behind which institutional patterns, not domestic ones, persist. A further problem is to be found in the perennial attempt to integrate the old people's home with its community.

But, to date, organic links are rare and community integration generally remains no more than a reflection of locality, the home being 'in' but not 'of' the community.

The key to unravelling these complex relationships will be a greater understanding of the day-to-day implications of the balance between dependence, independence, and interdependence for older people in residential settings. Focusing on the lives of residents and staff within publicly provided old people's homes, we have set out to discover how it is that the very act of becoming a local authority resident appears to disempower older people. We enquire whether the effects of institutional living exacerbate this dependent status; we consider recent innovations in care practices, and we try to assess the progress towards developing a liberal philosophy, and the effects that this may have on residents and staff. In so doing we confront this crucial question: can residential care offer a setting where the push and pull of independence and dependence give way to a form of interdependence, where resident, relatives, and staff can share the responsibilities for exchanging care in a way that offers mutual satisfaction? We suggest that residential settings require a substantial restructuring which will recognize, ameliorate, and perhaps resolve these contradictions and ambiguities upon which residential life is currently founded.

The magnitude of this undertaking cannot be overstated. And an important task for anyone who writes about residential settings must be to convey to the reader in a powerful way the strangeness of the set of arrangements that prevails in institutions in comparison with normal taken-for-granted patterns of living that we all share 'out there' in the community. Hence, before we embark upon a description of particular old-age homes, and the people who live and work there, we feel drawn to present a set of arguments which are based upon simple empirical data that have been conceptually fashioned to throw light on the physical and emotional distance that necessarily exists between, on the one hand, accepted traditions of family lifestyle and familiar associations of neighbourhood and domesticity, and on the other, the unusual situation presented by a group of erstwhile strangers living together in an artificial community, whose mores and social relations are ill-defined. We begin with a discussion of residential living.

Residential lifestyle

The concept of lifestyle tends to be physically located in the places where people reside; where they work; or where they spend their leisure-time. Varying degrees of activity or passivity may occur in arenas that are variously public or private. Individual lifestyle is thus determined by the particular configuration of circumstances that colour the daily round – and indeed, this is intimately linked to factors such as gender, class, race, and age groupings. For some, but by no means all, older people, lifestyle may be characterized by an emphasis on private and secluded participation in chosen activities and pastimes, and this tendency may increase with advancing age and greater frailty.

This preference for privacy may be the inevitable consequence of the fact that presently the majority of the 'very' old, people over eighty years, live in their own houses in the community and over half of these live on their own. The rest live with relatives: a spouse, siblings, and sons, daughters, and their families. Interestingly, hardly any elderly people live with non-relatives; only 2 per cent of those aged between eighty and eighty-four years and 5 per cent of those aged over eighty-five years have non-relatives in their households (OPCS 1982). In other words, access to private space, either in their own home or that of their family, is the typical expectation of very old people in Britain today. Hence the shift to residential living with strangers is essentially alien and may demand substantial adjustment from a group which is ill-equipped to respond.

The ideals for residential life have been defined as personal control of the living environment, a continuation of links with community, and, to use the official language of the last Building Note, a form of care which is 'domestic as befits function' (DHSS and Welsh Office 1973:5). The term 'domestic' is assumed to possess universal significance, yet in the residential context it must be shaped by special requirements which may conflict with traditional domesticity. It is therefore not an easy or comfortable enterprise to move beyond the simple rhetoric of 'domestic as befits function' to the practicalities by which the desired transformation is to be accomplished. We might pause to pose two questions: First, what is the nature of the domesticity being invoked by the Building Note and by those in the residential world who constantly use the analogy of home to explain caring practices and life in an old people's home? Second, is it possible to transfer traditional domesticity to the residential setting in whole or in sufficient part to justify continued use of the term?

There has never been any real challenge to those who write policy documents; in practice, therefore, the metaphor of domesticity has been extensively employed in the residential context, with the result that an old people's residence is construed as home. But the metaphor starts to break down when the distance between home in its traditional sense and home in a residential sense becomes too great.

In this text we present evidence to show that the residential version of home is considerably removed from the traditional domestic setting and, moreover, that domestic nomenclature does not rest comfortably within the residential setting.

The tradition of home

It should not surprise us that ideals of domesticity and of family are employed in the construction of residential ideals since the concept of home assumes a range of forms, and functions successfully across diverse cultures (Rapoport 1977). The suggestion that using the term 'home' to describe the residential form may not be legitimate implies that certain essential conditions of the domestic are not present in old people's homes. In order to justify this proposition we need to consider the nature of this traditional domesticity, and then to compare it with the residential variety.

Home has been conceptualized as having three dimensions: the physical, which relates to objects, spaces, and boundaries; the social, involving people and their relationships and interactions; and the metaphysical, which is the meaning and significance ascribed by individuals and communities to home. At the same time, home has been seen as having both a core and a periphery, the core being the dwelling itself which is conceived as the centre of an area called 'home range' (Downs and Stea 1973). This area within which the home is located is that physical space which an individual habitually uses – and within which people feel secure and in complete control.

The relationship between home and home-range or neighbourhood is symbiotic in the sense that each supports and gives meaning to the other, but at the same time they are distinct entities marked by boundaries. The boundaries of home serve not only as markers and defences by which strangers are distanced but also as membranes through which social exchanges become possible. Within these boundaries the individual or group expects to exercise control and outsiders are not expected to violate this area by assuming control. Moreover, control over a home environment is facilitated and expressed by the occupiers' psychological identification with the place. People adopt attitudes of possessiveness towards objects and their arrangement, and personal or group sense of identity is fostered in this way (Ittelson *et al.* 1974: 144).

Within the defensible space of home, the related concepts of territoriality and privacy apply. Indeed, one of the main consequences arising from territoriality is the establishment of a place where privacy becomes possible. Privacy is a complicated concept, but a broad definition is Westin's (1967) which suggests that privacy can be summed up as the potential for both concealing and revealing certain information about oneself. In one's own home it is secured tangibly by shutting out the rest of the world.

Domestic privacy clearly rests upon both social and physical factors. The boundary which distinguishes home from the outside world is one of the physical markers of privacy, but within this boundary other markers operate which reinforce and allow more subtle elaborations of privacy. This leads us to consider the physical structures by which home in its domestic sense can be recognized, the ways domesticity is expressed, and how it functions in terms of bricks and mortar.

Home, since it is the locus of living activity, must accommodate the basic tasks of daily living; it is made up of space for living. That distinct spaces are allocated to particular tasks – for instance, kitchens for cooking, laundry areas for washing things, bathrooms for washing people – is not simply an arrangement which facilitates domestic functioning. It is also an allocation, a spatial investment, which varies according to culture, class, and generation and which is a statement, and then a reinforcement, of the categories by which daily living is framed.

Certain kinds of allocations and juxtapositions of spaces appear to typify 'home'. Lawrence (1982) suggests that, whereas in newer houses dining is likely to take place in a combined dining-and-living area, in the older housing stock, typically occupied by older generations, eating is associated with a combined kitchen-dining area. We also know that some elderly people adapt the spaces in their homes so that sleeping spaces are at ground-floor level and may be combined with living spaces in ways which would not have been countenanced at younger ages when frailty was not a consideration. These are just two examples of improvizations made by certain groups upon domestic custom, but they suggest a control over home which may serve to enhance personal power in that a part of the environment is brought into line with the individual's particular needs and preferences.

We can argue then, that in our society, where the elderly are concerned, home is likely to be characterized by its enclosed and private nature since it shelters only a few, related people of similar generations. It is likely to be small. Whilst accommodating those activities necessary to sustain daily life, physical standards are unlikely to make life particularly easy for the elderly, who typically occupy the poorest housing stock (Hunt 1976).

This account of what might be entailed by the term 'home' for the elderly cannot claim to be comprehensive, since surprisingly little detail is available about older people's use of and attitudes towards the settings in which they live. Yet authors such as Harris and Lipman argue strongly that the relationships between people and architectural space are not simple and deterministic (1980). They entail complex interactions between people and the spaces and objects they use, and with their associated meanings. It is to this last topic, significance or meaning, that we now turn our attention.

The meaning of home for older people

The observation that home is of considerable importance to most people, but particularly to older people, is one that few would take issue with. It is a statement which reflects the ideal of family living to which society subscribes. But the reality is that many older people (and, indeed, people of all ages) do not live in family units; many live alone. Nevertheless, expectations concerning home appear to be important to old people and this is generally expressed as the wish to stay put (Wheeler 1982). What this suggests is that for most older people home has a psychological and metaphysical significance over and above being a shelter in which to conduct everyday living.

In such a situation, not only is there the obvious functional value of having a pool of potential help at hand, but there is the more expressive value of having links or connections with a wider society through traditional social networks. In many respects, however, this gives an over-optimistic image of old people as embedded in and connected to such networks. For many, such links will have been eroded by environmental changes and social and geographical mobility among their younger relations. And even those connections which are extant may have been weakened, if not exhausted, by demands arising from the frailty of older relatives and neighbours.

Yet one might argue that even old people who appear to be unconnected with their immediate settings, who may lack networks, and may seldom go out into the neighbourhood, *do* retain interests and connections with a wider society in which they no longer physically or socially participate. Given that access to other potential connections with society such as education or employment is restricted for older people, home will represent, for many, the one remaining domain through which they can connect with the wider context. In other words, home is a base from which older people can continue to engage in exchanges; it is a personal power base and a source of self-identity (Howell 1983).

Within the privacy of home, an older person can control, and often conceal, declining capacities in the management of daily living. The familiarity of the setting permits what Rowles calls a sense of 'physical insideness' where familiarity, at a less than conscious level, can compensate for the progressive sensory loss that is likely to accompany age (1983). The ability to continue to master the physical environment despite frailty confers power upon the individual, and this in turn can enhance personal capacity to interact beyond the locus of home. Moreover, such abilities will reinforce an older person's confidence to manage.

In another sense, the privacy experienced at home makes it possible for an older person to conceal incapacities and limitations from others who are sometimes only too ready to infer that incapacity in one area means incapacity across all areas of life. It is, however, an indictment of social relationships that older people should feel obliged to mask partial frailties for fear of being judged totally incapable of managing daily life. In reality the majority do remain at home until the end of life, and this suggests that partial frailty can be managed within the privacy and familiarity of home. So declining powers are buttressed both by physical and cognitive factors deriving from a familiar and controllable home base. For reasons such as this, it can be argued that older people are reluctant to leave homes which may be inconvenient and difficult, for to relinquish home would be to relinquish a hold on a base from which personal power can be generated and reinforced.

In this situation, what happens to home as a power base when privacy is attenuated by the need to bring in help for certain tasks? It might well be argued that home-helps and neighbours intrude upon that privacy in which frailty might be concealed and that as a consequence the notion of home is eroded. Whilst it might be said that where constant attendance and service are required, an elderly person's control of his or her home has been removed, it is also true that in the many cases where home-helps and neighbours give varying amounts and kinds of assistance, the older person retains significant territorial control and that privacy continues to characterize home. In such instances, neighbourly intervention can be negotiated and, in any case, home-helps invariably 'intrude' for only a proportion of the day and the elderly person retains a degree of control over access. But, perhaps more importantly, cognitive control is maintained. Even when a person is bed-bound at home and where considerable assistance by others is required, cognitive control of the environment remains within reach. In a known setting, metaphysical 'access' to other parts of the home persists, as do links to the memories associated with the home and the objects it contains.

The home experienced by elderly residents in care is, of course, organized on a much larger scale than that traditionally experienced in the community. However, many practitioners and policy-makers would claim that, apart from scale, the essential nature of home can be preserved in the residential home. We will present evidence to show that the residential form of home may be qualitatively different from the domestic home known to old people. It is our task in the following chapters to elaborate upon this argument; here we simply suggest that the residential home is different since it is arranged physically and organizationally to be public and, in such an arena, the control and concealment of frailty permitted at home are no longer possible. The reverse is true; frailty is revealed and exposed, with the consequence that personal power is diminished, so that the residential setting cannot be seen as offering a power base from which older people can engage in real, social and material transactions with others.

It is within this context that we now move on to lifestyles in 100 local authority residential homes. We describe a group of older people who have been obliged to relinquish aspects of privacy in favour of the public arena; a group whose temporal control over activities or passivity may be interrupted by the urgency of dull routine. Our study records the valiant efforts of residents and staff to resolve these contradictions.

The National Consumer Study of 100 public sector residential homes

This research was commissioned by the DHSS (Works Division) in 1980 and first reported in 1982 (Willcocks *et al*. 1982a). The main aim of this cross-sectional study was to evaluate those aspects of the residential care process which influence consumer satisfaction amongst elderly residents, with particular attention paid to the contribution made by the physical environment. The study was designed to meet the following objectives:

1 To assess the reaction of elderly residents in local authority homes to their present environment and to interpret the practical implications this may have for planners and architects; in particular, to generate material appropriate to a revision of Local Authority Building Note no. 2.
2 To determine the ways in which the quality of life experienced by residents may be influenced by a range of factors relating to physical environment, institutional environment, and resident mix.
3 To explore the attitudes of old people to residential care and to identify any consumer preferences or aspirations for environmental improvement which may exist amongst the elderly.
4 To investigate the attitudes and experiences of staff in residential homes for the elderly and to assess the impact of physical features

within the home environment.

5 To determine the importance of locational factors and the extent
   to which the convenience and proximity of the homes to local
   services and accessibility to family and friends may contribute to
   social and psychological well-being for both elderly residents and
   staff.

A full report on both the main findings of this study and its detailed
methodology is given elsewhere (see Willcocks *et al*; 1982a, 1982b). The
data reported in this text build upon those earlier findings, extending
our analysis and argument rather than replicating them. A brief outline
of methods used is given in Appendix 1. However, it is important to
stress that as this was a consumer study attempts were made to gain
several perspectives on the residential process. To this end, whilst the
main investigation involved interviews with 1,000 residents[1] and 400
members of staff in a representative sample of 100 local authority homes
for the elderly, these survey data were complemented by related studies
in a sub-sample of three homes: an observation study examined social
interaction patterns and the daily routine within homes; a location study
used mapping and field-study techniques to explore the relationship
between residential homes and the local environs. This multi-method
approach was deemed fundamental given both the complexity of institutional environments and the powerlessness of residents which often
manifests itself in the compliant responses to questions concerning
satisfaction with their current settings (Peace, Hall, and Hamblin 1979;
Booth 1983). The findings reported here draw upon the many data sets
gathered during the course of the study, mixing the views of residents,
staff, community members, and policy-makers with our observations
of the residential process. In this way we are able to contrast stated
policy with actual practice, highlighting the differences between them
and attempting to explain these contradictions.

The contradictions of caring

Our assumptions concerning residential care for old people are founded
on the history of past caring and our understanding of how that history
has shaped current practice. A consideration of this legacy forms the

basis of the first section of the book in which residential care is reviewed. Here we argue that certain features of present-day homes perpetuate the traditional and negative image passed down from Victorian times in which a harsh and custodial form of care was used to punish and stigmatize social outcasts. In this way we can begin to understand the residential home as an institution beneath the surface rhetoric of domesticity, and to see where the traditional struggle between the need to contain and the need to nurture has its origins.

Given the trends and arguments outlined in this first section, we are then in a position to revisit residential care and consider the current reality. Chapters 3, 4 and 5 focus our attention on the residents, the staff, and the physical world in which they live, and through a series of descriptions we begin to identify the sources of conflict within the caring process.

An initial discussion of the characteristics of residents leads into a wider examination of the process of becoming a resident and the gains and losses of residential life for those in need of some level of physical or social support. Here we find evidence, not only of the importance of residents' lifestyles prior to admission, but also of how the transition to residential status subtly changes the power of individuals, undermining their individuality.

This metamorphosis is facilitated by the residential staff, for although the residential home provides a living environment for residents it also provides a working environment for staff who are seen as the 'creators of care'. In Chapter 4 therefore we focus both upon the ways in which the caring task is constructed and on the characteristics of the individuals who undertake this task, their explanations for working with this group of elderly people, together with the degree of satisfaction that different workers achieve in residential practice. In discussing the caring task we demonstrate how organizational practices enable staff both to contain and nurture residents. We consider the possibility of resident-oriented or staff-oriented practices, and the kinds of lifestyles possible for residents in each setting.

Although the behaviour, attitudes, and actions of residents and staff form a major focus of the study, special attention is also paid to the physical settings in which these actions take place. Chapter 5 offers a description of the physical world of the old people's home, considering the range of buildings currently being used and describing the standards of provision, their amenities, and how design can affect resident privacy, safety, and manoeuvrability. Here we begin to understand the public/private divide in which both residents and staff act out their daily lives. Thus the built environment offers support to the contradictions in caring and, whilst we do not espouse architectural determinism, we acknowledge the trend to find built solutions to social problems. Thus consideration is given to how the physical environment is used, and whether residential homes are designed primarily with the needs of residents or staff in mind.

Following the variety of insights into the residential process described in Chapters 3–5, in Chapter 6 we attempt to draw this wealth of material together within one framework, which is discussed within the context of a review of the major contributions to theory in this area. At the outset of the National Consumer Study a simple model of the residential process was proposed. Thus it was hypothesized that within the institutional setting three main areas would have a direct effect upon resident well-being: the physical environment, the institutional environment, and the resident mix. These were defined as follows:

1 *Physical environment* – the internal and external world of the home, for example design and layout of rooms; the ratio of single to shared bedrooms; the relationship between the home and its external surroundings.
2 *Institutional environment* – the levels of independence maintained by residents; areas of resident choice and decision-making; the level of structure and rigidity which may characterize home routine; the extent to which residents can achieve a satisfactory degree of privacy.
3 *Resident mix* – the characteristics of all the elderly people using the homes either as permanent residents, short-stay residents, or day-attenders, for example their age/sex distribution, and levels of physical and mental impairment.

Subsequent secondary analysis of the data sets, supported by ESRC,[2] increased our understanding of the complexity of this process, and has allowed for the extension of this model as outlined in *Figure 1*. This has resulted in further definition of the institutional environment to include both aspects of organizational structure and regime,

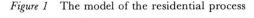

Figure 1　The model of the residential process

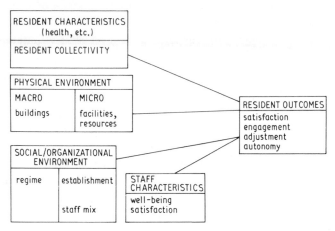

the addition of staff characteristics, and the differentiation of macro and micro resources within the physical environment, as well as a greater cross validation of data sources (details concerning the scope of secondary analysis are given in Appendix 2).

In Chapter 6 we extend this attempt to understand the residential process by trying to answer the following questions:

1 Can we distinguish a range of residential environments in terms of the lifestyle offered to residents?
2 If so, do some residential environments enhance resident well-being more than others?
3 Can residents perceive an 'ideal' supportive setting which can be compared to the realities of residential life?

In focusing on these questions, consideration is given both to the range of physical characteristics and organizational practices within homes, and how such variation relates to both resident and staff well-being. Special attention is paid to those homes in the sample which incorporate small group living, as an example of the most recent innovation in care practice. By seeking the answers to these questions we try to establish whether or not it is possible to settle the conflicts between containment and care, private and public lives, independence and dependence which we suggest are common to residential life. Finally, the views of residents elicited through the 'visual game' technique are considered and conclusions are drawn concerning the wishes of residents for an environment that is seen to be 'normal, non-exceptional, non-institutional', where they experience a level of environmental control.

Having revisited the residential setting, our task in the final section of the book becomes one of re-ordering and seeking a resolution to the contradictions in care. Chapter 7 outlines one innovation, based on the concept of a 'residential flatlet', although it is argued that such a design solution must not be adopted as a panacea for all residential ills. The case is made that any alternative constructed upon design alone will fail unless it is accompanied by an acknowledgement that there is a proper role for residential care, in the spectrum of service, which is not merely a default option where community care breaks down. Such an acknowledgement should lead to a massive restructuring of residential provision involving changes in the attitudes of residential staff and other professionals working with the elderly, as well as in the wider community.

The concluding chapter focuses specifically on this 'unfinished business' and seeks a solution to the task of empowering older people, both within the residential setting and in the world outside, for it is important to widen the debate beyond the immediate concern with the lives of those who live and work in homes. At the risk of being labelled 'residential determinists' we suggest that a re-evaluation of the principles underpinning residential options can provide a practical focus for raising critical questions concerning the future role and form of social welfare, and ways in which it might be shaped by the consumers of care to enhance their own quality of life.

Notes

1. Within the resident interviews resident preferences for aspects of the physical environment were elicited through the use of a visual game technique which overcame some of the problems of institutional socialization (see Willcocks 1984).

2. Secondary analysis of the data was supported by the ESRC (Ref. G00232019) and through ILEA research fellowships.

CHAPTER 2

The legacy of past caring

Any discussion of policy and practice in residential care must recognize the challenge of a new era in which growing old is no longer experienced as a novel social event. Substantial numbers of frail dependent people aged seventy-five or more are now making their legitimate demands on the state (Blythe 1979), and these increasing numbers and legitimate demands have to be seen against a backcloth of national economic difficulties together with social and political change. This, *inter alia*, has encouraged a shift in focus towards the provision of community care which is often regarded as a preferred and lower-cost alternative to residential care (DHSS 1981a; 1981b).

Over the past decade, residential care services have come under increasing attack from a number of sources. Critics on the right deplore the inefficiencies of investment in institutional provision and they claim, correctly, that at best it will benefit only a minority of those in need of care. Critics on the left present evidence of breakdown within the institution and argue that old people's homes have failed to provide a successful challenge to the historical and cultural echoes of the Poor Law. Indeed, it is fair to point out that much of the current public debate concerning residential care has tended to concentrate on issues of cost-efficiency, as in the work of the Audit Commission (1985), with relatively less concern being addressed to the more problematic areas of effectiveness. Accordingly, the best efforts of policy-makers and caring professionals across the political spectrum have been directed towards community provision – arguably to the detriment of residential care services.

This chapter will explore the material circumstances and the ideological commitments that have given rise to this crisis of confidence in residential care for old people. This will involve a consideration of the historical role of the workhouse in Victorian society, the change of political philosophy which is associated with the dramatic shifts that have taken place in the design and organization of homes in the forty years of the Welfare State, and the massive changes foreshadowed by late-twentieth-century demands for a restructuring of welfare – and a return to the Victorian values embodied in Poor Law provision. We will argue that historical developments have failed to confront the essential contradiction between the care and control aspects of institutional provision. Furthermore, much of our present difficulty in re-ordering residential settings, and introducing progressive policies which acknowledge the rights of old people to exercise choice and control within institutional settings, can be seen to derive from attempts to resolve current social problems with a practical formula that is both inappropriate and underdeveloped. Essential characteristics have been inherited with only minor adjustments from a nineteenth-century model which was designed to incorporate fear and repression.

An appropriate starting-point for this discussion is official policy on old-age homes which finds expression in the National Assistance Act, 1948. This requires local authorities to provide 'residential accommodation for persons who by reason of age, infirmity or any other circumstances are in need of care and attention which is not otherwise available to them'. Different forms are used to translate this policy into residential practice but essentially the old people's home has been society's way of managing that residual group of elderly people who cannot manage for themselves. And we can argue that this represents a form of social control that can emerge in different modes at different historical periods. Its form is sometimes overtly repressive, sometimes paternalistic. It was originally designed to limit the demands of older people upon the state and it serves to emphasize the marginality of the old, the poor, and women in the different stages of a developing capitalist society. This of itself suggests that community care must inevitably represent a better option for old people. But a realistic appraisal of the life and times of the older generations and the circumstances that delimit their social horizons in late-twentieth-century Britain might lead us to ask: 'How much better served are those old people who live in the community?' The balance between independence and a supportive environment and the different ways in which this might be achieved either side of the present residential divide will be a theme which recurs throughout this text.

A century of Poor Law provision

In order to understand the relationship between old people and the state it is necessary to return to the origins of statutory residential care which lie with the Poor Law amendments and the development of indoor relief and the workhouse system (Peace 1983). To obtain support or benefit the Victorian claimant was obliged to submit to the workhouse test under which homeless, rootless, and penniless individuals were required to enter an institution which would provide minimum sustenance in return for work. It is clear that the early industrialists deliberately created institutions which would punish and stigmatize indigents.

According to one Assistant Commissioner of the Poor Law the object was 'to establish therein a discipline so severe and repulsive as to make them a terror to the poor and prevent them from entering' (Townsend 1981: 8). Thus was the work ethic stimulated, and social deviants including the elderly poor were punished for transgressing conventional social norms. The Poor Law asylums were constructed as mass establishments for several hundred inhabitants apiece; they were intended to provide a harsh regime of custodial care, where conditions were spartan and overcrowding was the norm. They were designed to house all of those whom society had rejected. In this way a social and physical separation developed between those who came to be regarded as the deserving and the undeserving poor, and in accordance with the principle of lesser eligibility it was important to demonstrate that a miserable fate could be anticipated by all those who failed to heed the warning of the workhouse (Pinker 1971).

Despite the unattractiveness of this solution, many thousands of elderly people were obliged to enter these institutions and at the turn of the century some 115,000 were obtaining relief in this form. It is undoubtedly true that the workhouse model evokes fearful memories which can threaten the potential resident amongst the current generation of older people. The reform of the workhouse system, or public assistance institutions (PAIs) as they came to be known, was slow in coming. In 1939 there were still nearly 400 public assistance institutions, accommodating 149,000 residents, 60,000 of whom were classified as sick (Ministry of Health 1939) and it was not until the massive social movement that took place in the period of the Second World War that any substantial change in policy occurred with respect to accommodation for elderly people.

In the critical period of change in social relationships signalled by the Beveridge Report of 1942 there were a number of precipitating factors which contributed to the push for institutional reform. First, there was a need to discharge patients from existing hospitals in order to accommodate war casualties; this meant that many frail and sick elderly people were forced either to seek admission to a public assistance institution or to fend for themselves. Second, many elderly people living in large cities were made homeless due to air raids. And third, the culmination of these events led to the overcrowdings of PAIs. This in turn resulted in the development of evacuation hostels by government and voluntary organizations as a response to the plight of the homeless (Means and Smith 1983). At a more fundamental level, this was to become the era of massive social transformation as Beveridge targeted his five loathsome giants – want, idleness, squalor, ignorance, and disease. He produced a framework within which universality of social security could operate, and for the first time there was anticipation of the kind of pension that would remove deep-rooted fears of poverty in old age. At the same time, social policy in the areas of education, health, and social services provision was establishing the principle of equality of opportunity together with equality of access to a range of supportive services – from the cradle to the grave.

This was to provide the historical moment for voluntary organizations to undertake a substantial review of the kind of institutional solutions that had been attempted in the past and to devise alternative care programmes for initiating change in accordance with the social democratic promise which inspired the post-war planners. They began to make the case for developing small hostels which would be purpose built and designed to accommodate the infirm elderly; these hostels might be regarded as the forerunners of today's small modern home. As part of this process, growing criticism of PAIs through the Nuffield Survey of 1947 paved the way for implementing post-war reform on the basis of a move away from the harsh, communal, mass establishment where privacy was non-existent towards the domestic scale of the hostel which begins to address the needs of the individual resident (Nuffield Foundation 1947).

This seemingly radical proposal emanating from the Nuffield Survey Committee was that old people who are no longer able to live an independent life in their own homes should be accommodated in small homes of thirty to thirty-five beds, and not in large institutions. Furthermore, it was envisaged that such provision could be assured, primarily, through state intervention in association with the voluntary bodies. Thus alternative ideas around residential care for old people were entirely consistent with the social democratic philosophy promulgated by the post-war Labour government and enshrined in reports and legislation across a wide range of social welfare issues. Indicative of the degree of change that was envisaged is the radical suggestion that the old 'master' and 'inmate' relationship endorsed by the workhouse should be replaced by something akin to that of hotel manager and guest. This dramatic change was codified by the National Assistance Act, 1948.

Post-war policy changes

What is particularly notable in the early post-war period is the attempt by policy-makers to control the physical structures of institutional provision. There is less evidence to suggest a concern with the normalization of lifestyle within the home. During the early 1950s a norm of thirty to thirty-five beds was encouraged and a substantial level of building followed, but by 1955 a government review indicated that sixty might prove a more appropriate size to cater for the increasing numbers of infirm residents and to meet the needs of organization. This subsequent reversal towards a more institutional form proved unsatisfactory, to residents and staff alike, and in 1962 revised guidelines appeared in the form of a DHSS Building Note (DHSS and Welsh Office 1962).

This document was the result of more than a decade of state intervention which had witnessed the disappearance of many former workhouses and a decline in the numbers of adapted properties. It did make positive recommendations concerning the advantages of community integration; it noted the limitations of isolated greenfield sites and it warned against developments which might create elderly ghettoes. In terms of interior design it made recommendations on room size, level of amenity, and personal furniture, all of which were intended to promote a domestic home-like image. At the same time, in his classic study of residential care published in 1962, Townsend was able to demonstrate the persistence of certain workhouse traditions and he revealed traces of the old Poor Law which permeated the new welfare institutions (Townsend 1962). And we must record that few homes built during the 1960s were able to achieve a strict adherence to those ideas advocated by the 1962 Building Note.

In the absence of a fundamental rationale for old-age homes, beyond the general exhortation contained in Part III of the 1948 Act, it was unlikely that any radical revision of the nature of institutional care could take place, for it remained severely underconceptualized. Nevertheless, in an attempt to deal with various problems at a symptomatic level a process of reform was initiated. And so a series of ad hoc developments started to transform the face of residential caring. In some homes, separate units were developed and these could be adapted, in some cases, for the needs of the elderly mentally infirm, and in 1967 the novel concept of short-stay care was introduced, which marked the beginning of the multi-purpose home (Ministry of Health 1968, Allen 1983).

In 1973 a revised Building Note provided a more detailed account of the physical world of care and acknowledged some of the more progressive elements in old-age homes that had begun to appear (DHSS and Welsh Office 1973). It codified the notion that homes should be 'domestic as befits function' and addressed the complexities of residential life that emerge in relation to the needs of different user groups: the introduction of day care, short-stay care, and a meals service in the multi-purpose home, the desirability of greater community integration and the need for residents to achieve privacy and self-determination, as well as enhanced personal security. Recommended scale was between thirty and fifty beds; facilities and room size were to be increased and for the first time the concept of group or family unit design was advocated – a device which incorporates both architectural and organizational features in the endeavour to reduce the mass scale of institutional living arrangements.

The 1970s also witnessed a growing anxiety about the future of 'an ageing population' and in 1978 the Labour government produced a discussion document, *A Happier Old Age*, which suggested that due to the increased demand for residential places local authorities could be asked to provide more beds within a reduced capital programme (DHSS and Welsh Office 1978). Gradually the changing economic climate and a shift in the nature of ideological commitment to social welfare paved the way for a marked withdrawal from state supported residential care.

The change in attitude towards the frail and vulnerable is perhaps best encapsulated through the titles and themes of official publications. There is a sense of alarm conveyed by *The Rising Tide* (Health Advisory Service 1982) which warns of a substantial increase in the numbers of elderly people suffering from mental infirmity at the same time as suggesting a service response, and the Conservative government's white paper, *Growing Older* (DHSS 1981b), which takes us into the 1980s and establishes the ground rules for a substantial diminution of state intervention around the provision of care services and care networks. This latter document states clearly that community care offered by family, friends, and voluntary organizations will provide most of the services required by most old people. The failure of the social democratic promise is complete and the monetarist language of self-help, thrift, and responsibility (values attributed to the early Victorians) is promulgated in order to encourage old people and their carers alike to buy their welfare in the market-place.

Contradictions persist, however, insofar as the 1981 white paper does approach the issue of quality of care – not with respect to a recognition of entitlement to social welfare from childhood, through one's work-ing life and beyond, into retirement as conceptualized by the post-war visionary policy-makers but, instead, as a response to consumer demands. In the case of residential services there is an explicit demand by clients and their carers for a more caring and homelike environ-ment; this is supported by the demands of service providers for a more efficient service that would be cost-effective and custom-made for the more dependent members of the elderly community. Within the context of the market-place, where goods and services are exchanged, the relationship between the provider and customer constitutes the main focus of interest. Accordingly, the intention to carry out a consumer study of residential services was announced in the white paper. It was in this context that researchers from the Polytechnic of North London were commissioned to investigate the design preferences and aspirations of elderly residents in relation to local authority homes (Willcocks *et al.* 1982a, 1982b).

Historical trends in building design

We have already seen that the historical development of public sector residential homes has been contained within a particular ideological framework and that since 1948 there has been an attempt to espouse conflicting agenda, the provision of care, and the need for 'containment'. In terms of building design this has resulted in two competing interests. The first concerns the desire to create for old people deemed to be 'in need of care and attention' a homely domestic setting which maintains vital links with the community. The second concerns the viability of maintaining institutions for so-called marginal groups in society and this has tended to produce the rationale for pursuing economies of scale. The tension created between these two aspects of policy is evident.

While the adaptations of large domestic houses and small hotels allowed for the growth of small homes in the 1940s and early 1950s, as we have noted, the need to accommodate greater numbers of frail residents led to the development of larger purpose-built homes. The recommended size of homes was to settle finally between thirty and fifty residents as outlined in the 1962 Building Note and its subsequent revision in 1973. However, while very large homes were now to be avoided, only homes with more than thirty residents were seen to be economically viable.

'The Department supports the view that in a home of more than fifty places it is difficult to sustain a domestic atmosphere and considers that normally homes should not exceed this size . . . A balance of economic and other values suggest a home of between thirty and fifty places . . . The capital cost per place of homes for less than thirty may rise sharply.'   (DHSS and Welsh Office 1973: 3)

Yet the importance of financial constraints lies in direct contrast to the architects' concern with creating an environment that captures something of the domestic setting. It has been demonstrated that, since 1948, architects have been concerned to move away from design features that are seen to be overtly institutional, for example, long corridors and multiple bedrooms, and to utilize features associated with domestic architecture (Barrett 1976). However, as a result of the need to maintain a certain number of residential places, architects began to focus on the size and importance of the living unit, rather than on the size of the building. This led to the development of the group unit design which paralleled the desire amongst policy-makers to recreate the family unit within care settings.

This idea of self-contained units was introduced in the 1962 Building Note and was discussed in a number of articles in *The Architectural Journal* during the 1960s and early 1970s (Korte 1966; Goldsmith 1971). Korte recommended that where her suggested optimum twenty-five residents was exceeded, then the number of residents in a home should be limited to approximately forty who were accommodated in family groups of some eight individuals. She also proposed that a majority of residents should be accommodated in single bedrooms and that if possible a WC be provided either for each room or shared between two bedrooms (Korte 1966). The concept of family groups was to be supported in the 1973 Building Note, and developed further by both Barrett (1976), and Lipman and Slater (1977a), who proposed a design where bedsitting rooms, incorporating a separate shower/WC room and lobby, covered an area of approximately 25 square metres. In reality, however, the purpose-built group unit design homes built in the 1970s commonly accommodated forty to fifty residents in five groups of eight to ten people who each had his or her own bedsitting room but shared a small communal eating/dining area and bathroom facilities. In 1980 the present study estimated that a third of local authority homes were operating some form of group living system, not necessarily purpose built.

It is apparent, then, that a move away from the institutional past of workhouse design to a more domestic style has been given support both by independent architectural observers and in government publications. However, as we shall see, the domestic analogy may be difficult to operationalize, given aspects of scale, function, and interpersonal dynamics. The importance of such trends can be seen in the wide variation in the types of residential home found within the National Consumer Study. Importantly this evidence comes from a representative stratified sample of 100 homes in England in 1980. The investigation revealed that more than four-fifths of the homes included in the study had opened as residential homes for the elderly since 1960; 75 per cent were purpose built and the remainder were based in converted properties, half of which had modern extensions. Almost 50 per cent of the homes accommodated forty to fifty residents, although numbers ranged from thirteen to eighty-two. Whereas seventy-seven homes were run on fairly traditional lines, twenty-three homes incorporated some form of group living arrangement. They included eleven homes where residents lived in small groups and twelve where a mixture of group and communal settings were combined – these homes are referred to as semi-group homes. The degree of variation suggests that socio-historical influences and different professional approaches over time to the design and organization of residential environments will have a profound impact on the daily experiences of those who live and work in today's old-age homes.

The development of care concerns

At the same time that questions were raised about the relationships between institutional design and lifestyle, additional policy issues were being addressed through parallel research activities. A particular concern for policy-makers and service-producers has been appropriate placement for the frail or confused elderly, and appropriate levels of service support. Official guidance has traditionally proposed that different types of accommodation should be purpose designed for different categories of old people. Those whose physical health necessitates continuous medical or nursing care should be cared for in geriatric wards, those suffering a degree of mental illness or infirmity which warrants medical or nursing care should be placed in psychiatric or psychogeriatric wards, and the remainder whose condition does not warrant special health care but who are unable to live unattended in the community should be cared for in residential homes. The role of nursing homes in statutory care for old people has yet to emerge (Atkinson, Bond, and Gregson 1985).

Research in Manchester by Evans and colleagues looked at the mix of lucid and confused residents in non-specialist residential homes for elderly people (1981). They found that the capacity to provide satisfactory care for heavily dependent residents is determined primarily by the level and quality of support staffing, and speculate that a typical residential home, if adequately staffed, might cater for 30 per cent confused residents without adverse effect on the working lives of staff – and the residential experiences of those who live in the homes. In part, the study is located in that unhappy professional clash between the medical and social work models of care and the advantages of social service settings as opposed to hospital settings for the long-stay elderly. Subsequently, in a comparative study of four different sectors of care, Wade *et al.* (1983) revealed a remarkable degree of overlap in the profile of client dependency. Elderly people in geriatric wards, psychogeriatric wards, residential homes, and those living in the community were compared. The researchers concluded that undue attention has been focused on appropriate placement for old people even though this has demonstrably failed to achieve a homogeneous population within the different sectors. Indeed, it is obvious that client needs shift over time and controlling the characteristics of clients in a given environment will prove problematic for service-providers and clients alike. They argue that policy should focus instead on providing appropriate supports for a broad range of client needs in all settings.

Essentially these two studies suggest that we have allowed arguments about where old people are placed to obscure the important issue of securing adequate and flexible resources that will enable the very frail and confused to be properly cared for in whatever sector they may be located. This suggests that a more sensitive use of community nursing care and ancillary support services plus a complement of peripatetic care staff could enable a residential home to receive additional support during periods of increased dependency amongst the residents and, importantly, where frailty decreases, or on the death of heavily dependent clients, services could be withdrawn. In part, this emphasis on moving clients between services reflects the significance of those artificial constructions that operate in a relatively autonomous and professional manner within the rigid boundaries of the service divisions. Health workers and social workers have not permitted joint planning or joint financing exercises seriously to erode their independent mode of operation, and, perhaps of greater concern, within social services departments the residential workers and staff working in area teams may have occasion to meet only in situations of crisis or conflict. Collaboration in client care under these conditions, both within an agency and across different authorities, will remain a pious aspiration in in the absence of structural change. A pragmatic response to client need will inevitably tend to generate a move across boundaries rather than a reappraisal of alternative methods of providing services to that client within the sector in which he or she happens to be located.

Much of the rigidity in thinking which might be said to characterize the different service-providers located securely within their own sector must be attributed to the isolation of the different modes of the care network one from another. This in itself is largely determined by a series of historical, legislative, and organizational accidents. Of particular concern is the gulf which exists between official policy and practice on community integration. Over the years a series of uncoordinated policy documents on the organization of institutional care and the design and location of homes has advocated practices which aim to promote and develop meaningful links between the home and the community (Willcocks 1986). Policy statements refer to the siting of homes and advocate locations which are convenient for local shops and amenities. They note the requirement of residents to visit post offices, and perhaps the church or the pub, as a way of sustaining important links with normal everyday activities. Equally important is the need to select a location that facilitates visiting by family or neighbours who remain in the community. This suggests that physical proximity, an absence of slopes and inclines, or a good bus route should be foremost in the planner's mind. However, evidence from the National Consumer Study suggests that locational factors are inappropriately defined in relation to the reality of community integration.

A second aspect of developing community links is to be found in those policies which advocate the use of resources associated with residential settings to provide a range of different services for the community. The concept of the multi-purpose home is one which might appear very attractive to the hard-pressed service manager who seeks to maximize capital and labour investment for the broadest range of needs within the client group. Hence the development of homes which can offer short-stay respite care, for rehabilitation purposes or to help caring relatives; some homes will extend their catering services to provide a meals-on-wheels service, or more usually a luncheon club for visiting elderly people; entertainments provided in homes might offer a welcome diversion to the isolated elderly in the community; and it has become commonplace for the homes to offer some form of day-care, although the scale and regularity of such provision varies widely.

Evidence from the National Consumer Study suggests that there has been only partial implementation of strategies such as these among local authorities. Indeed, there are problems arising from the different requirements of designing and organizing an establishment to evoke domesticity and homelike environment and one which aims to function as a resource centre. Conceptually and practically this issue has received insufficient attention from policy makers; initiatives have tended to be imposed by the specialist provider rather than developed organically from a community base. As a result, the multi-purpose home has made little impact on the traditional divide between the institution and the community at large. This is perhaps not surprising given that governments have generally developed their policies for the residential home quite separately from policies for the community, thus creating and perpetuating within the DHSS the traditional division in which community care is simply represented as activity outside the walls of the institution while life within the institution is perceived as beyond the boundaries of community care. Such a philosophical distinction is then expressed in practical terms by the manner in which local authority services are primarily designed and managed as discrete entities to support a particular group of clients in the different sectors. Thus social critics, with justification, will continue to describe residential homes as socially marooned (Townsend 1981) for they observe that the physical walls of the institution have been reconstructed as policy categories.

The separation of residential care from community care might well be justified in terms of administrative criteria relating to the efficient distribution of limited resources to those deemed eligible for a particular service. Yet evidence suggests that this argument may be founded upon a rationality which does not exist in practice. We have noted that it can be both ineffective and inappropriate to design discrete services for client groups with allegedly different needs since the actual distinction between the groups is largely an artificial one (Wade, Sawyer, and Bell 1983). And there is wide professional agreement that a more satisfactory alternative involves the flexible adaptation of services to client needs and closer collaboration between the various options along the care spectrum.

Much of this separation which we describe and which elderly clients experience has a history which is deeply rooted in the harsh nineteenth-century tradition of relief, where little distinction in terms of treatment or accommodation was made between the poor, the sick, the insane, and the criminal. The question this raises is to what extent present-day institutions can challenge this negative image through the development of alternative material and organizational forms in the late-twentieth-century residential home. We might experience some doubt if we refer to Goffman's treatise on the total institution (1961) which is conceptualized on the basis of features which include the routinization of daily activities, together with formal rules and block treatment of clients around a rational plan designed to meet the aims of the institution. Such an environment serves to dehumanize the individual and may prompt pathological reactions such as withdrawal from participation in everyday activities (Barton 1966). It would be dishonest to deny the persistence of such features in our present-day homes.

This suggests that there remains much in the spirit of the institutional environment which limits opportunity for communication and interaction with the outside community – thereby reinforcing barriers from the past. Geographical isolation in large buildings plus an artificial sexual or social segregation of clients and staff typify patterns of relationships which evoke an earlier period. Furthermore, for the newcomers there is the strange encounter with the special language of residential life; they learn terms like 'superintendent' or 'officer-in-charge'; there are unfamiliar routines such as 'toileting', together with rule-bound notices to residents; and there are demeaning modes of address like 'gran' or 'luv' plus distinctive home names. All of these constitute the deep-rooted traits that mark out the home as an institution.

We do not encounter this nomenclature nor these various insignia in the 'normal' world experienced in the community. It becomes viable and legitimate only in situations where external social controls are imposed as a means of securing institutional goals. Thus we label and give identity to a separate group of people and we construct a boundary around them which can deter the most committed and caring outsider from venturing across the threshold. In this way, ideological distancing has been reinforced by the material form that creates a separate dimension of care.

Yet as we seek to challenge this isolation under the social democratic umbrella of welfare provision in the 1980s we encounter further problems which derive from the deliberate confusion which has been created around the term 'community'. It has been suggested (Tinker 1984) that a narrow definition of community care might mean the provision of domiciliary as opposed to institutional services, while an alternative view presents an ill-defined cosy picture of a group of local people caring for their neighbours. In reality, the impetus for community care has been shown to lie within a broad framework in which the anti-institutional lobby looms influential (Johnson *et al.* 1983). At the same time, there has been a political shift, prompted by the need for economic restraint, away from statutory services as providers of care, in favour of a model whereby statutory services support and enhance the caring capacity of the voluntary and private sector.

> 'money may be limited but there is no lack of human resources. Nor is there any lack of goodwill. An immense contribution is already being made to the support and care of elderly people by families, friends and neighbours and by a wide range of private, voluntary and religious organisations. We want to encourage these activities so as to encourage and develop the broadest possible base of service.'
>
> (DHSS 1981b: iii)

The manner in which this is to be achieved remains unspecified – and deliberately so.

Unfortunately this has resulted in a dysfunctional and dangerous opposition between a programme for community care which remains unclear in its conceptualization and residential care which is usually presented as being rigid and isolated. The very fact that community care policies have this blurred image must seem attractive and gain credibility when juxtaposed with the inflexibility of residential care. This haphazard historical opposition has become deeply rooted in our attitudes to care alternatives and it tends to colour the way in which society endeavours to protect old people from the harsh fate of a residential future. There is an entrenched defensiveness about the way in which residential care is offered to clients and nowhere is this more evident than at the point of cross-over into the residential sector.

The legacy of past caring, then, is to create a sector which, at a macro level, repels outsiders by its strangeness and inaccessibility in terms of known forms of care and familiar patterns of living. It can also be argued that the evolution of care to its present form is such as to encourage a conceptual split between institution and residential home. This is reinforced by the knowledge that workhouses have been eliminated. There then follows a reluctance to scrutinize the activities that constitute residential living in the modern home and to admit the possibility that remnants or transformations of institutional practice – if not policy – may persist. As a consequence modern residential practice may preserve aspects of history which work against reform.

CHAPTER 3

Crossing the threshold

In order to understand what residential care means to old people, it is important not just to consider the characteristics of residents but also to examine the process of becoming a resident and the relationship between the nature of admission and the successful adaptation to a new environment. The prospect of moving into an old people's home is seldom viewed with pleasure; indeed we suspect that most old people, even of advanced age, keep such an option out of mind until perhaps a particular change in circumstances forces such a consideration. The impressions that older people have of residential life, if not entirely coloured by images of the workhouse tradition of the past, are often based upon some knowledge of the restrictions that will be placed upon them. Old people's homes may be thought of as suitable for some old people, but not for themselves. For many, too, the residential setting is seen as a place to die, and the acknowledgement of this fact is often experienced in stark contrast with the old person's determination to survive. Moreover, events prior to admission will have a significant impact on the subsequent construction of a resident's life once relocated in the home, for, although institutional factors will influence this outcome, they are not the sole determinants of the way residents cope with the change to residential life.

There is a history of investigations into the process of crossing the threshold into institutional care, and professional opinion generally concurs that deleterious effects may be associated with the actual transition into care. This should not surprise us, perhaps, given that admission represents a unique event for the elderly person; he or she is walking away from a life in the community, which has a history that can be traced back over some eight decades, in order to enter a place where the future may be measured in weeks or months, just a few years at best. If we accept that the happiness of old people in a residential setting, their behaviour, and their well-being, is the combined product of the characteristics of the institution and the process of relocation, then it behoves us to question the pathways and procedures that lead to residential care. This in turn raises vexed questions of choice and control in later life which are so frequently denied to people once they are identified as clients.

Relocation from community to care

To date, studies of the relocation of elderly people from their homes in the community to institutional settings have shown that such moves are, for many, disadvantageous, resulting in increased morbidity and mortality and a decline in both activity levels and psychological well-being (Lieberman 1961; Blenkner 1967). Importantly, it is not just the change of environment and the impact of adverse institutional effects, but the extended process of relocation itself that is seen to be stressful. In this context, few researchers have separated process and outcome, relying in the main on cross-sectional studies of old people already admitted to a residential home and comparisons with community samples. The present study is no exception, and because of this limitation it is important to consider the circumstances surrounding admission. The work of Tobin and Lieberman (1976) is particularly important in this connection. In introducing their longitudinal study of applicants to three homes for the aged, they outline a number of factors which may affect the well-being of residents aside from the traditional institutional effects. First, selection bias – whether particular types of people, who may be more vulnerable than others, enter care; second, pre-admission effects – that is the adverse effects of becoming institutionalized prior to entering and living in the institution; and third, environmental discontinuity, the loss associated with moving, which they suggest may vary depending on the degree of discontinuity between the two environments:

'The larger the difference between the new and old environments – with expectations being equal – the greater the possibility that the elderly person will need to develop adaptive responses beyond his capacity.'   (Tobin and Lieberman 1976: 20)

They go on to suggest that such factors, along with the effects of institutional living, are not necessarily mutually exclusive. The portrait of the elderly resident must be viewed in terms of a wider perspective which encompasses the period of time from the decision to seek residential care, through the period of waiting to enter the institution, and on to the initial adjustment phase of the first two months in care and the survival of the first year. Their empirical study, which rests upon comparisons between community, waiting list, and resident samples, as well as on a longitudinal study, demonstrates that the effects of institutionalization begin prior to admission. Those on waiting lists and those in care are more alike in terms of cognitive functioning, affective responses, emotional state, and self-perception than those in the community sample – a process confirmed by the longitudinal study. While our present study lacks the data necessary to confirm these findings, this cannot be ignored in our analysis of the impact of institutional effects upon residents; indeed it is fundamental to our discussion of the characteristics of residents and the lives that they lead.

Additional information on difficulties around admission emerges from a new study of 550 applications for Part III accommodation in an inner London borough (Lawrence, Walker, and Willcocks 1986). Evidence is presented of the uncertainty and lack of control for the older person that characterizes the period following the completion of a formal application for residential care. Three months after the date of applications 52 per cent of applicants were actually living in an old people's home, 10 per cent were in a geriatric ward (of whom two-thirds had been there at the time of application), 2 per cent were in a psychogeriatric ward, and 2 per cent were in sheltered housing; just over a fifth were living in the community. Of all these a third had been in hospital at the time of application and although most were still awaiting Part III admission some were said no longer to require it; one in ten had died over the three-month period (some after moving into a home), and there was a handful who went into a home but did not stay.

Is there evidence of selection bias?

In 1962 Townsend commented that residents in local authority old people's homes 'differ markedly' from elderly people at large (Townsend 1962: 59). But are residents unrepresentative of their age-peers in the community? The average age of residents in our study was eighty-three years for women and seventy-nine years for men, with 82 per cent of the sample over seventy-five years of age. Comparisons between those older people living in the community and those in care should therefore be made amongst the very old. Census data show that over two-thirds of the population over seventy-five are women; in care 73 per cent of those sampled were women (OPCS 1983). The pattern is not dissimilar. What is true, however, is that a greater proportion of female residents was found amongst those over eighty-five years of age as compared to older women living in the community.

If we consider the impact that these variations have on actual numbers of residents in an average forty-bed home, then the age/sex differences appear more dramatic. *Figure 2* shows that in the 'young' old categories there are twice as many women as men (sixteen and eight respectively), but in the 'old' old category there are four times as many women as men (thirteen compared with three). Such variations may have important consequences for the kinds of services that these different groups of old people may require and their expectations about residential life. Further, we would suggest that the presence of substantial numbers of very old women may have a determining influence on the way in which members of staff perceive residents as a whole and this in turn may affect the way staff relate to residents.

Amongst younger residents a large percentage was divorced, separated, or never married, and therefore predominantly without the support of children or spouse (*Table 1*). Of male residents over seventy-five years, the number of widowers increased dramatically. This confirms not only the traditional association between bereavement and the need for support (Townsend 1962; Smith and Lowther 1976), but also that elderly men are seen to be ill equipped to carry out the domestic tasks necessary to remain in the community, a view revealed in the attitudes and actions of service-providers and relatives (Hunt 1976; Finch and Groves 1983). The absence of married couples

Figure 2 Age–sex distribution of residents for a typical forty-bed home

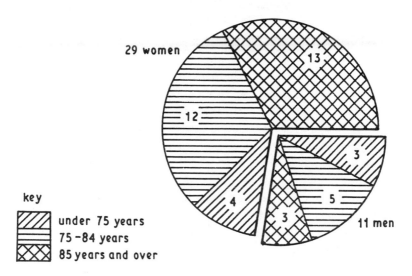

29 women

key

under 75 years
75 –84 years
85 years and over

11 men

within care settings also confirms the support a spouse provides; 4 per cent or thirty-eight of the residents in the sample were married and only half were living together in the same residential home. While there may be a variety of reasons why married residents lead separate lives, it is also true that homes lack the facilities which would enable the privacy of married life to be maintained (Hughes and Wilkin 1980).

Table 1 *Marital status of residents compared to 1981 Census data (%)*

	60–74 years				75 years and over			
	Sample		Census		Sample		Census	
	M	W	M	W	M	W	M	W
married	5	5	76	44	6	4	61	20
widowed	36	61	14	42	71	75	30	64
divorced separated single }	58	34	10	13	23	22	9	15
N = 100%	73	106			186	593		

Sources: Willcocks *et al.* (1982a) and OPCS/Registrar General, Scotland (1983).

Almost half of our sample of residents had been living alone prior to entering the residential home. While this proportion is not unusual for women in their late seventies and eighties, comparison with census data shows that for men the numbers who had been living alone were disproportionately high, highlighting their deviant marital status (OPCS 1983). A comparison of residents' length of stay in the home with previous residence shows that in recent years more residential places have been taken by those living alone than those living with other relatives. It seems reasonable to suggest that a connection exists between the increase in the 'very' old population, shifts in the domiciliary services for the elderly living alone, and the persistent expectation that caring relatives will continue to bear the burden of support for aged relatives.

Residents were also likely to have been living in another institutional setting, a hospital, or other old people's home, prior to admission – a finding supported by other studies (Evans *et al.* 1981; Wade, Sawyer, and Bell 1983). For these residents environmental discontinuity has already taken place and research has shown that hospitalization can affect an older person's decision to move into residential care. Sinclair and colleagues in their study of applicants to local authority homes found that those from hospitals were much less likely to change their minds about an application to residential care, the break with the community having already been made and the process of institutionalization already being underway (Sinclair *et al.* 1983).

Finally, little is known about the social class of residents in local authority homes or the variation in social status of residents in different types of residential settings. Along with other studies, the present research has failed to overcome the difficulty of assessing social class for older people in care, whose current lives bear little relation to their former position in or outside of the labour market. Because of this we must acknowledge that differences in socio-economic status may exist; indeed those with the financial resources to purchase alternative forms of support or care obviously have more scope for choice than do those who must rely solely on state provision.

Our analysis shows that there is some evidence of selection bias amongst residents, but that this is particularly true of younger residents and male residents. The characteristics of 'very' old women, who form a majority of residents, are similar to those of old women living in the community. This group, rather than being perceived as deviant, may simply be those who have survived beyond the limits of their community support. All of these factors point to the importance of social circumstances in influencing admissions, and support the suggestion that the old person newly admitted to residential care may be characterized by one or more of the following features: aged over seventy-five years, single, childless, living alone.

Choice, control, familiarity

The main reason given by residents for their admission to residential care was a reduced ability to manage in their own domestic setting. This was attributed to a number of factors including the immediate consequence of an accident, a specific period of poor health, and a more generalized decline in the capacity to perform the tasks of daily living. Sinclair and colleagues comment that 'the factors which lead to an application for residential care do not develop suddenly' (1983: 3), and case histories from their study show how an accumulation of problems, including bereavement, failing sight, increased houseboundness, unsuitability of present housing, can lead to a situation in which it is difficult for the elderly person to maintain life in the community. Given these circumstances a single event such as a fall can result in admission.

While many of these older people will have been living alone, others will have been dependent on an ageing spouse, family, or friends. Problems associated with caring family or friends accounted for approximately one in five admissions in the present study; an inability to cope or a breakdown in care accounted for 20 per cent of male admissions and 15 per cent of female admissions. In many cases a chain of events culminated in a situation where caring relatives could no longer cope, as the following example shows: 'I was living on my own: I kept falling. I'm blind and I couldn't manage. I lived with my niece for a short time but then she was ill. I came here for two weeks and I just stayed on.'

Reasons for the breakdown in caring relationships include the increasing frailty or ill-health of the care-giver, especially common where the relative is an ageing spouse or sibling; problems associated with competing responsibilities to different family members which can result in conflict; and the increasing strain on carers which the practical, social, and emotional pressures of the relationship may bring, particularly where the old person is mentally frail (EOC 1982; Sinclair *et al.* 1983; Levin, Sinclair, and Gorbach 1983).

A small percentage of residents in the present study attributed their admission to bereavement and, given the number of widowers, it is not surprising that this explanation was more common amongst men. The explanation of one male resident was not uncommon: 'After my wife died my doctor said I couldn't stay on my own.' The intervention of third parties – doctors, social workers, and other professionals – is obviously of critical importance in influencing the decisions of many old people and their relatives. More than one in five respondents gave reasons for admission which we have termed 'unsolicited arrangements by GPs, social workers, or other agencies with whom the resident has been involved in their previous setting'. The fact that so many old people reported so little control over their admission to care is disturbing and gives some indication of the process whereby individuals are disempowered.

In contrast, we must also mention the group of residents who make the decision to move to a residential home in a fairly rational way, believing that it may be the best course of action for themselves and their families. While it is, no doubt, true that some residents will overclaim that the decision to enter care is their own, adopting this coping strategy in order to avoid recognition of rejection by their family and society, we would also suggest that where residents do make a positive choice it can be rewarding: 'I hadn't been well and felt alone. I chose this home because I played the piano and I can practise every day. I have my own room and it is surrounded by gardens.' This explanation reveals not only the desire for companionship, but also a knowledge of the home and the expectation of both personal privacy and the continuity of past activities – all positive factors which may ease transition and adjustment. Given the importance of these decisions, having prior information concerning the residential options available in the locality and being able to exercise a choice, may be the key determinants of future well-being.

The relationship between choice, familiarity, and control are crucial to our arguments concerning the nature of private lives in public places. Becoming a resident in a local authority home involves the transition from community living to something which is unfamiliar and about which the individual has little choice. At the time of admission only 38 per cent of respondents in our study had made a prior visit to the home. Furthermore, it appears that alternatives were also limited; only one in five was given a choice between the home he or she actually entered and other possible establishments. Such findings undoubtedly reflect the hurried nature of many admissions, a genuine lack of resources, and the direction of different residents to particular homes. Yet, in spite of this general lack of choice and control, there is evidence that certain reasons for admission, for example bereavement – which particularly affects men – or the family being unable to cope, are seen by residential staff as more legitimate than others. Such legitimizing can affect the transition to care and the way residents adapt to communal living. Indeed, those with legitimate reasons for moving were more likely to have been offered a choice of homes, to have visited their new residence, and to have brought with them to the home a range of possessions from televisions to small pieces of furniture. As a result of this we discovered them to be less prone to homesickness, more likely to make new friends, and better able to interact with staff.

Familiarity and choice are also linked to the availability and accessibility of information concerning the range of residential alternatives available in a particular area and what to expect from residential settings. Since the consumer study was undertaken, and certainly since our respondents became residents, there has been both an increase in the amount and availability of private residential care and an increase in information about residential options and lifestyles (Wilson 1984; Kellaher, Peace, and Willcocks 1985). Such developments may begin to enable older people and their carers to make more informed decisions about their future long before a crisis emerges.

The health of residents

Discussion of the social factors surrounding admission to residential care highlights the variety of circumstances which older people may experience. Although a decline in health plays a primary role, as we have seen, poor health alone provides insufficient cause for admission. Furthermore, the overall level of dependency of residents in care may result from a number of other intervening policies concerning admission to care. Studies have noted the wide variation in the level of residential provision from one part of the country to another (Darton 1984) and how this, along with the availability of a range of alternative services, may affect admission policies and resident selection. The design of homes may also have a bearing on selection, especially where homes with several storeys or without a lift impede mobility. All these factors taken together will therefore influence the level of physical or mental functioning displayed by residents in any one home, and the range of ability or disability will have an effect on the lives of residents as individuals, as a group, and on staff.

In order to assess residents' levels of functioning in the present study, senior staff completed the Crichton Royal Behavioural Rating Scale (Wilkin and Jolley 1979) for each resident included in the stratified sample across the hundred homes. However, owing to the difficulty in obtaining complete interviews from 31 per cent of the original sample, a system of substitution had to be introduced (see Appendix 1). Substitution was due to three main factors: mental infirmity (53 per cent), ill-health at the time of the interview (15 per cent), and deafness (13 per cent); only 7 per cent refused to be interviewed. Details of the overall distribution of the Crichton Royal scores for both actual and original samples are given in *Table 2* and show that the actual respondents were less mentally frail and more capable of caring for themselves than was the original sample.

Some idea of the variation in levels of disability amongst residents can be noted in individual items of the scale. In terms of mental frailty, between 14 per cent and 34 per cent of the original sample were classified as showing some signs of infirmity on the five dimensions of mental status. These figures, although not directly comparable, are within the same range as other studies in local authority homes. Thus Charlesworth and Wilkin (1982) found 41 per cent of residents moderately or severely confused, and Booth *et al.* (1983a) found 28 per cent mildly or severely confused. Such findings indicate that the mentally frail form an important minority group within homes. Such a comparatively small group can make disproportionate demands on staff time, which may account for the over-estimation often made by staff that a large proportion of residents are mentally confused. Of course, aspects of physical health such as incontinence can also place a particular burden on staff. The study found that 43 per cent of residents were not fully continent, a figure comparable with the 41 per cent found in the study of homes in twelve local authorities carried out by the Personal Social Services Research Unit (PSSRU) in 1981 (Bebbington and Tong 1983) and 35 per cent in Booth's study of four authorities (Booth 1985). Of those who were incontinent, 6 per cent were doubly so – a small percentage but a group which again demands a disproportionate amount of physical care from staff. Yet, while some residents had particular problems in terms of self-care, most could dress and feed themselves without assistance. Only with bathing were most residents offered help, a finding which perhaps tells us as much about staff routines as about resident ability.

While mental frailty and double incontinence affect a small group of residents, mobility problems are more commonplace; 55 per cent of the original sample were said to be fully ambulant or usually independent while 35 per cent walked either with an aid or with supervision and the remaining 10 per cent were chairfast or bedfast. In contrast to other areas of functioning where the actual sample interviewed were less frail than the original sample, mobility problems were more comparable, and further analysis of the actual sample shows that women particularly suffer in terms of mobility and that these difficulties increase with age; 35 per cent of female respondents over eighty-five years of age used walking aids. When asked about the use of aids, women were more likely to use zimmer frames or sticks, while men predominantly used sticks. Our observations also showed that the use of frames was in some ways more handicapping than the use of sticks; they were rarely used outside the home, being bulky and difficult to transport, and additionally conveyed a rather more prosthetic image.

Changes in health over time

In recent years much has been written concerning the increasing mental and physical frailty of residents within residential homes. The validity of this assessment has been questioned and recent work by Booth and colleagues has challenged the myth of rising dependency, highlighting the deficiencies in cross-sectional studies which present only a snapshot

Table 2 Distribution of Crichton Royal Behavioural Rating Scale – giving age–sex distribution for actual and original samples

	original sample %	actual sample %	(actual sample) under 85 years men %	women %	85 years or more men %	women %
mobility						
fully ambulant/usually independent	55	60	71	55	70	41
walks with supervision	9	6	7	9	5	11
walks with aids	26	27	14	26	21	35
chairfast/bedfast	10	7	8	10	4	13
memory						
complete memory/occasional forgetfulness	69	85	82	68	80	60
short-term loss	10	8	7	9	11	12
short-term and long-term loss	21	8	11	23	9	28
orientation						
complete/oriented within home	66	81	82	66	73	56
some misidentification	17	13	11	18	18	19
can't find way to bed or toilet	7	4	3	7	3	10
completely lost	10	2	4	9	6	15
communication						
always clear/can indicate needs	85	96	88	86	92	79
can't understand simple information or can't indicate needs	4	1	5	3	2	7
can't understand simple information *and* can't indicate needs	5	2	4	4	3	6
no effective contact	6	1	3	7	3	8
co-operation						
active/passive cooperation	75	86	77	75	86	71
requires frequent encouragement	16	11	14	16	8	19
rejects assistance/ill-directed activity	4	2	6	4	3	4
completely resistive or withdrawn	5	1	3	5	3	6

Table 2 *contd.*

		998	999	201	408	68	318
restlessness	none/intermittent	86	93	88	85	89	86
	persistent by day or night	4	3	5	4	0	4
	persistent by day *and* night	5	3	2	7	5	4
	constant	5	1	5	4	6	6
dressing	correct/adequate	68	80	77	66	85	60
	adequate with some supervision	13	11	9	15	5	15
	needs constant supervision	10	5	7	12	5	11
	unable to dress/retain clothing	9	4	7	7	6	14
feeding	correct unaided	79	88	86	79	86	72
	minimum supervision	16	9	12	16	8	21
	needs continuous supervision	3	2	1	3	5	5
	requires feeding	2	1	1	2	1	2
bathing	washes and bathes unaided	9	13	18	8	13	5
	minimum supervision	35	43	44	34	47	27
	close supervision	26	26	20	26	20	32
	continuous supervision/requires bathing	30	19	18	32	20	36
continence	full control	58 }	70 }	89	85	92	80
	occasional accidents	27 }	21 }	2	4	2	8
	continent if toileted	5	3	4	6	3	4
	urinary incontinence	5	3	5	5	3	8
	regular/frequent double incontinence	6	2	5	5	3	8
	N =	998	999	201	408	68	318

of resident dependency at one point in time (Booth *et al.* 1983b; Booth 1985). Comparisons between the PSSRU 1981 survey and the 1970 DHSS Census of Residential Homes show that there has been an increase in dependency levels during the decade, especially in the group classified as moderately dependent (Bebbington and Tong 1983). However, while it can be accepted that changes have taken place over a ten-year period, such analysis does not tell us anything of the variation in type of resident dependency and the complexity of fluctuations over time. Booth's longitudinal study of dependency in four local authorities during the early 1980s revealed no significant difference in the levels of overall dependency during the three years (1985). However, this general stability represents the cumulative effects of movements into and out of care, masking the enormous turnover of residents over time. Of the 6,947 residents included in their census in 1980, almost two-thirds were absent from the 1982 census, and of this group 66 per cent had died and 21 per cent had been transferred to hospital. Whereas the most severely dependent residents were those most likely to die during the two years of the study, there was no trend towards increasing dependency amongst newcomers (Booth 1985). Booth's study is important because it points to changes in the resident population over a relatively short period of time which have a direct bearing on staff working practices. Thus staff have to cope with a high turnover in residents, as well as fluctuations in the type of dependency. A severely mentally confused resident who dies may therefore be replaced by someone who is doubly incontinent; both may be assessed as heavily dependent but make entirely different demands on the workforce. The study also indicates that almost a quarter of residents were assessed as independent on all measures of dependency used and, in following up a sample of sixty-three very independent residents, Booth notes the importance of the pathway into care and suggests that a proportion of old people could manage outside the residential setting (Booth 1985). The residential home therefore caters for those who need a great deal of physical care and those who need minimal support, a fact which obviously presents staff with a conflict in terms of the organization of caring practices.

Table 3 shows the distribution of Crichton Royal scores for physical impairment and mental frailty for the thousand residents by length of

Table 3   *Crichton Royal scores by length of residence and sex**

Length of time in care	Original sample		Actual sample	
	physical	*mental*	*physical*	*mental*
under 1 year	5.6	4.9	4.6	3.3
1 year	5.8	5.2	4.5	3.3
2–4 years	6.1	5.0	4.4	2.7
5–9 years	5.3	4.4	4.5	2.6
10 years or more	4.0	4.1	2.7	2.3
x̄	5.7	4.8	4.4	
male	4.2	3.5	3.5	2.3
female	6.2	5.3	4.7	3.2
x̄	5.9	4.8	4,4	
maximum score	19	19	19	19

**Note:* A detailed account of this scoring system is given in Willcocks *et al.* 1982b.

residence and sex. Scores are calculated on a scale from zero to nine-teen, where nineteen represents maximum frailty. Comparisons of the original and actual samples show that female residents are more mentally and physically frail than male residents, although overall scores are low for all residents. There is no strong pattern in relation to length of residence. Indeed, given Booth's findings, we should guard against over-interpreting cross-sectional data. What is apparent, however, is the low scoring achieved by the small sample of respondents who have lived in care for ten years or more, which may be indicative of differ-ing circumstances surrounding admission during the early 1970s and is reflected in the high levels of functioning of these survivors. Varia-tion in the mental and physical health of residents and the proportion of residents at any one time who are seen to place heavy demands on staff will have important implications for both how staff view their role and the ways residents are perceived as a group. It may lead to more or less emphasis by staff on physical care and the perception of residents as a dependent group.

Well-being and satisfaction

It is clear from our discussion so far that the feelings of well-being or satisfaction reported by residents reflect not only their present circumstances, but also an accumulation of events which encompass their life in the community as well as the process of admission to residential care. Because of this, it would be unwise to attribute all negative feelings of well-being to the effects of institutional living.

Residents' psychological well-being was assessed with a modified version of the Adjustment to Ageing Scale developed by Abrams and first used in a study of the community elderly (1978). The scale consists of three positive and four negative statements which respondents are asked to consider as true or false (see Appendix 2). It attempts to measure how well or badly older people feel they have come to terms with growing older. Abrams, using a ten-point scale, found that for a community sample of people aged over seventy-five, those living alone were far less well adjusted than those living with others; this tendency was more marked amongst men. In our institutional sample, no noticeable trend occurred for the whole sample, with a fairly even distribution centring on a mean score of 7.6. Further analysis revealed that men (7.9) were slightly more adjusted than women, and higher scores were also recorded by those long-stay residents whose physical (7.8) and mental (7.9) health was above the median as measured on the CRBRS scale and the small group of residents (N = 24) under sixty-five years of age (10.4) who were nearly all resident in an old people's home owing to some physical disability which demanded a degree of care deemed unavailable elsewhere. In addition to considering the scale as a whole, the individual statements provide descriptive data of intrinsic interest. The first statement – 'all your basic needs are taken care of' – was overwhelmingly agreed upon by 94 per cent of residents, with little variation between different groups of residents. However, slightly more women than men claimed to be 'miserable most of the time', and this was particularly true for female newcomers (25 per cent as compared to 11 per cent for males). More women than men felt that they 'no longer do anything that is of real use to other people' (47 per cent and 36 per cent respectively), and again this was particularly acute amongst most recent residents. The feeling of uselessness and that everything was done for them was very prevalent amongst residents. A substantial proportion of respondents also failed to establish more than casual acquaintance with other residents in the home. One-third of the men and women interviewed 'no longer had anyone to talk to about personal things' and just over 40 per cent 'still felt lonely at times'. Close friendships between residents were rarely observed during the detailed studies, neither did residents discuss issues together other than superficial ones.

This indirect measure of well-being was complemented by a more direct approach at ascertaining current life satisfaction. Thus residents were asked: 'How satisfied are you with life as a whole these days?', followed by 'and before you came to live here?' A comparison of the two questions shows that 45 per cent of the sample maintained the same level of satisfaction.

Finally an attempt was made to examine the levels of anxiety experienced by residents, measured in terms of 'worries'. Respondents were asked whether, during the past few weeks, they had been worried about any of eight issues ranging from money and family to the way the home was run and their health. The measure was adapted from an instrument developed by Srole in 1962. Overall worry scores reflect the low anxiety recorded by residents, the majority scoring only zero or one. Little variation is noted for particular groups of residents although those who had been resident for ten years or more reveal particularly low scores. The main areas of concern focus on health (34 per cent) and the possibility of falling (33 per cent). At an earlier stage in the interview respondents had given a subjective self-assessment of their health and a majority had reported themselves as in good or fair condition. The worry item therefore tapped an underlying fear concerning health that in general was more apparent amongst women (36 per cent) than men (29 per cent). The difficulty which residents may experience in coming to terms with health anxieties is vividly portrayed by the woman who stated: 'In the last six months I have been losing weight and I'm worried in case I have cancer; no, matron wouldn't be interested – she says I look fit and well.' The way in which residential homes manage health care is a somewhat contentious issue (Bowling and Bleatham 1982) and staff attitudes may serve to heighten residents' anxieties, as indicated above. The fear of a possible fall was voiced by 25 per cent of men and 36 per cent of women, which reflects differences in mobility and use of aids noted earlier.

It is not surprising that family worries concerned almost a fifth of residents (17 per cent of men, 20 per cent of women). However, these anxieties declined with both age and the number of years in care, a pattern that was also seen in relation to financial worries. In the case of concern over money, this worried more men than women (16 per cent, 9 per cent respectively). In the case of both family and financial matters, a decline in anxiety no doubt reflects the distance residential care creates from previous activities and expectations regarding lifestyle.

The remaining items of the worry index concern aspects of home life. While only a small group of residents expressed anxiety over the way the home was run, of greater importance was the issue of safety; 9 per cent of men and 13 per cent of women were concerned about the safety of their personal possessions, and for women this worry increased with the length of time in care. Personal safety worried a higher proportion of the resident population; 18 per cent of men and 17 per cent of women were concerned about safety in the event of fire. This is an emotive subject about which strong responses are to be expected and will be raised again in our discussion concerning resident preference within the residential setting.

When asked if they had any worries about things not covered by the scale, three-quarters of residents said they had none and a typical response was: 'No, I don't worry at all, I've finished worrying.' For the remainder, issues relating to health were mentioned most frequently, together with comments relating to the ageing process, physical deterioration in general, and to some extent loss of role. One respondent commented: 'I have no worries, nothing except getting older and feeling I have lived my life now.'

While the individual items of such well-being measures are of interest in themselves, the composite scales indicate the variety of feelings expressed by residents about getting older and living in a residential home. Elderly residents are by no means a homogeneous group, and, even if there is some evidence of selection bias in terms of the circumstances precipitating admission, the responses to that admission are by no means uniform. The measures described here will be used later on in our analysis when we consider the effects of institutional living. First, however, we consider the reality of residential life for these old people.

Gains and losses experienced in the move to residential care

The ideal upon which residential life rests is the provision of care and attention to those for whom this is not available in the community. The price to be paid for such benefits is, however, a less commonly acknowledged aspect of the process of becoming a resident – for there are costs and losses as well as benefits and gains and it is this equation that an older person has to translate, in very personal and individual terms, if residential life is to be comprehensible. This is not easy, as the terms of the residential 'contract' are not often spelled out clearly. Nonetheless, as we have seen, a proportion of residents do manage to construct a personally coherent explanation as to why they made the move into care, and the observation study revealed that a small number of residents (about 10 per cent) organized their lives in ways which suggested they maximized the best that residential life had to offer and minimized the worst. Such residents would typically spend a lot of time in their own rooms, watching television, reading, or writing letters and in relative solitude, knowing that support was at hand if needed. That this group was not especially popular with care staff, often being regarded as stand-offish, is another indicator of the conflict in which staff are placed in meeting the dual goals of providing care and attention while nurturing ideals of independence.

This recognizes that there are at least two main parties to the agreement, their interests and values may not be identical but a *modus vivendi* has been constructed and the terms of entry can then be laid down in a formal agreement. In return for warmth, security, and a range of care services from the staff, the client agrees to give up some individual freedoms; however, in submitting to the plan laid down by the social services department he or she also forgoes rights and entitlements to other freedoms. Sadly, procedures such as these remain a rarity and going into care retains its pejorative image. It stays alien, different, and distanced from all other experiences which people accumulate over a lifetime.

Such issues of rights and risks where older people, especially those in care, are concerned have become the subject of discussion over the last few years (Norman 1980). The problem in the residential sector is that staff are charged by society with the task of protecting residents from the harms to which they are thought to be liable in the community. This is one of the rationales for making residential care available. It is the yardstick by which staff do their jobs, it is the justification offered to relatives and carers who can no longer cope, and it is the basis by which residents are urged to move from a relatively isolated domestic setting to a supportive residential community.

We have already seen that most residents agree that all their needs are taken care of. In certain respects this is an acknowledgement of the protective nature of residential care, and in some instances it also represents an insistence that this should indeed be the case, for residents enter care having been assured that they will have no need to worry about things like shopping, cooking, and looking after the house. It is at the point that older people become convinced that they can no longer manage such daily tasks that they acquiesce in the transfer to care. Thus, dependence is integral to the contract as far as the potential resident is concerned. However, there is a paradox here since, once in care, though the ideal of independence is put about, the practice cannot be encouraged since too many independent activities would disrupt the routines through which care is delivered.

The advantages of residential care in terms of support with everyday tasks are obvious enough. Residents are not concerned with looking after themselves or with cooking or domestic tasks. Financial aspects of their accommodation are dealt with and property maintenance is no longer a problem. There is very little of a material nature that concerns residents, and this will be a relief to many who have struggled on alone. On the other hand, the frameworks which structure ordinary daily living in the community are no longer available to residents, and other ones must be developed. The course of least resistance is for residents to adopt residential routines and this is the most common response. This, however, encourages the block treatment of residents, leading to the ubiquitous apathy.

Thus, the uncertainty of life in a community environment which made excessive demands on an old person is exchanged for an environment which is routinized and predictable, often to the point that hardly any demands are made upon residents. This is a problem of residential life which exercises staff and policy-makers alike but which, for the most part, remains intractable. This is despite the introduction, in many homes, of modest cooking and catering facilities for residents or their visitors to use. It seems the case, however, that such additions to residential life are only cosmetic or token, and few residents organize their lives around the use of them. Thus, in many respects, the physiotherapy of everyday activity is lacking in residential settings.

A distinct advantage of the residential home is the superior physical setting in which the old person lives. Even when homes fall short of an ideal standard they can offer greater care and comfort than that experienced by an old person before admission. But against this must be weighed the loss of a familiar home which represents links with the past. All too often only tokens of a former home life can be accommodated in the residential bedroom. Similarly residential settings are generally less hazardous than the domestic ones older people are likely to have occupied. Few stairs, the existence of hand rails, and similar aids contribute to safer living. But these local authority homes are large buildings, often complicated in layout, and many residents, especially the women, admitted to not knowing the building and to rarely venturing beyond their particular patch. Thus, few residents are able to take advantage of their new and safer environment in terms of enhanced mobility.

One of the major problems for old people living alone is the anxiety – their own or that of neighbours or relatives – about the possibility of accidents. However, the removal of anxiety or risk through admission to a more supportive residential setting is inevitably associated with a corresponding loss of independence. The relief felt by older people and their relatives that, for instance, risk of fire, accidents, and isolation have been reduced, is undoubtedly accompanied by a recognition that some of the interest and unpredictability of ordinary life has also been removed. In its place is the unpredictability of one aspect of institutional life – the other residents. It is interesting to note that concern about the risks of fire breaking out was an issue placed high by residents in the visual game choices (see Appendix 1) they were asked to make. This suggests that the concern registered by the public, by policy-makers, and by staff as to the safety of residential homes is shared by residents too, and that they recognize quite clearly the special kinds of hazards associated with a communal style of living.

There is little doubt that in residential homes the health needs of residents will receive regular attention, the staff being constantly alert to the possibility that residents may become ill. Nevertheless, the health hazard of residential living is that frailty and confusion meet together under one roof and this can present an exaggerated impression of the ageing process which might distress individual residents, especially newcomers, and may lead to a lowering of morale among all residents.

In all, this adds up to greater physical safety for residents with a reduction in anxiety in certain respects. However, the residential attempt to eliminate the physical and emotional risks associated with isolation has, generally, resulted in a lifestyle for residents which is not the independent one which freedom from anxiety might bring about. Instead it is often a lifestyle constrained by institutional imperatives to organize the reduction of risk.

The process of becoming a resident, then, is one which for most residents is an experience of the environmental discontinuity of which Tobin and Lieberman write (1976). The minority of residents who had been able to exercise even a small degree of choice as to when and where they would go to live in care tended to make more satisfactory adjustments once in a residential home. For these few, we might argue that the discontinuity is less, simply because of the link forged between life in the community and life in a home by even a minimal amount of involvement in and control of the transition to care. For the others – the majority – these links are virtually severed and, as we have seen, the residential life is one which is quite unlike the domestic one in terms of routinization and institutional safety precautions. It is therefore very difficult, if not impossible, for residents to pick up the threads of everyday life in ways which have meaning for them if the connections between former community life and the new residential life are not preserved and nurtured as part of the admissions procedure.

The finding that so few residents could recall choice or discussion about their admission is testimony to the likelihood that institutionalization starts well before admission. That an older person acquiesces in such an important step as admission without exercising any real choice is, in itself, a capitulation, an admission of powerlessness which is part of a process that legitimizes those further erosions of self and independence we know as institutionalization.

CHAPTER 4

Creators of care: staff

It is only partly true to say that those who staff old people's homes are the creators of care since residents themselves contribute, by their presence and through their dependencies, to the exchanges which take place around the acts of giving and receiving support. However, having said this, it is the activity of providing care rather than the passivity of receiving it which comes across as the more 'creative' part of the process and it is, of course, the staff as a whole which is engaged in this undertaking. Here we consider both the ideals and the practice of caring in local authority residential homes and, having regard for the gaps which inevitably occur between ideals, policies, and practices, examine the relationships or connections between these parameters – for, while residents experience, in a very direct way, the consequences of particular practices, the influences which shape residential care may impinge only indirectly on residents' lives. To the extent that residents share with staff an appreciation of the ideals on which support is founded, it might be said that both parties create rather than collude in care.

The term 'care', like many others, is open to a host of interpretations and can be operationalized and find expression at a number of levels. It may be the case that the residential package is a restricted or partial one when compared with care provided in other contexts. Nevertheless we should consider the residential variety against broader and more general notions since these latter 'realities' contribute significantly to the ideology which legitimizes the rendering of care by staff to residents.

Probably the most pervasive ideals or models of care are those which occur within traditional kinship boundaries, especially the 'informal' care of children by parents. The kinship model is characterized by the all-embracing nature of care-giving. The carer is available twenty-four hours a day and the activities in which he/she engages are many. The range may cover those tasks necessary for physical survival as well as those conducive to the recipient's intellectual and emotional development. Such care is generally characterized by an integration of tasks so that emotional care is frequently locked into 'subsistence' care. Research in the residential sector (Clough 1981) suggests that the parenting ideal of total care is at least a part of the framework within which residential workers operate and, as Graham (1983) argues – though in relation to the domestic setting – the parenting care model is likely to be the mothering one.

But there are other models upon which residential staff draw. As Harris points out (1977), parents do not work a forty-hour week, have six weeks holiday a year, employ domestic help, or live in separate accommodation or, it might be added, draw a regular wage for the labours of love. The work model, and sometimes that of organized labour, comes into play here. Other models of care available to staff are the professional ones of medical and social work. Thus the roles assumed by those who care, and the corresponding ones adopted by the recipients of care, are shaped by several influences. But others are at work which should also be taken into account for an understanding of the significance of the residential caring task for staff and its impact upon residents. It is a fairly obvious fact that staff undertake care from a work-base which is hierarchic and organized in character, but the concomitant fact, that the staff working world is not the same as the resident living world, is not always recognized. Yet care and the currency – dependency – by which it is exchanged are associated with distinct domains, each having its own culture.

The staff group

It is important to see the staff 'team' of an old people's home in context as being part of an accountable social service department line management team. But, having said that, the group which works together within a particular establishment does so at a day-to-day level as a three-tiered structure made up of officers, care workers, and domestics. The stratification of these staff is a reality which is accepted unquestioningly by everyone involved, with each level of staff having a characteristic set of tasks.

Figure 3 *Distribution of tasks which make up residential care across different categories of staff*

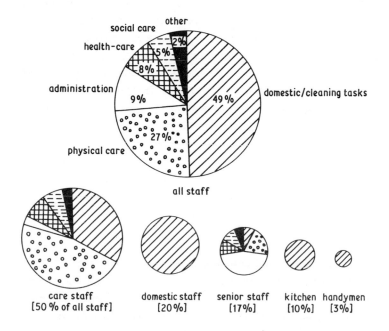

Other researchers (Imber 1977; Evans *et al.* 1981) have undertaken detailed classification of the tasks entailed in residential caring. The distinction between supervisory staff, care staff, and domestics which Imber makes is one which is reflected in our findings, though with Evans and colleagues we would tend to agree that night staff represent another distinct group. Additionally, we include kitchen staff and handymen in the following description of staff who, together in a particular home, deliver the care package to residents.

The heavy investment made in care staff, the accomplishment of domestic tasks about the home and the physical care of residents is shown in *Figure 3*. Taking account of all staff across the hundred homes, not just the staff sampled for interview, we find that half of the total contracted hours were allocated to care staff, with domestic staff absorbing a fifth of the hours available. Senior staff worked some 17 per cent of established hours, with kitchen staff taking up a fifth of the total time and handymen being employed for just 3 per cent of the total staff hours – although sixty-three out of the hundred homes employed at least one man to assist with maintenance inside and outside the home.

It is clear that care assistants carry the weight of the caring task, with domestic staff supporting them. For every three hours of care-staff time, there is generally one hour of supervisory time and slightly more than an hour of domestic support. Domestic staff were engaged mainly as part-timers working a weekday morning shift and in fifty-eight of the homes all domestics were employed on a part-time basis. Where care staff were concerned, only six homes had all care staff as part-timers; most homes had a mix of full-time and part-time care staff to cope with shift systems of working. In contrast, only 6 per cent of senior staff had part-time contracts and even this small group was contracted to work around thirty hours a week.

The corollary of these contractual arrangements is that care and domestic staff, already predominant in terms of total hours contributing to the care package, are also numerically the largest groups in terms of personnel. Senior staff, on the other hand, represent only 13 per cent of all the staff. These ratios of supervisory to care personnel, along with the hours invested at each level, have implications for the styles of care residents are likely to receive. It is from senior staff that ideas on new or more 'progressive' approaches to resident care are likely to emanate and, in theory, to be transmitted to care staff. We find for instance that senior staff hold more resident-oriented views on features of residential life such as the desirability of single rooms. Care staff are more likely to express views which spring from organizational needs for routine. Moreover, it is senior staff who benefit from training – either outside the job or in service – with the intention that they should spread the good word in their homes. The extent to which these goals can be achieved will depend, at least in part, on the time which senior staff can allocate to supervision of care staff. *Figure 3* shows that the greater part of a senior officer's time is absorbed by office tasks, thus limiting supervision time even further. Senior staff were conscious of the gap which could develop between themselves and care staff, but shortage of time often meant that supervision, in its broadest, supportive sense, became inspection, to ensure that worst practice was avoided.

If administration preoccupies supervisory staff, the physical care of residents typifies the care task. The categories of activities shown in *Figure 3* emerge from an analysis of staff responses to an open question. The categories correspond closely to those Imber isolated which also validated the now accepted nomenclatures of residential care, so that we find certain tasks clustered at different levels in the care team. Imber showed that the boundaries between clusters was not a fixed one (1977). In our study we also found a division of labour that, despite hierarchy and issues of status, was not entirely rigid. While domestic staff had a fairly clearly delineated set of tasks which centred around cleaning the home, for care staff the job was not so clear-cut. When domestics were not on duty it was care staff who did the necessary cleaning. Moreover, night care staff undertook a whole range of domestic duties, for instance cleaning lounges and tidying kitchen cupboards, and senior staff often undertook domestic and kitchen work when there were staff shortages. In one home, the deputy officer in charge replaced an absent cook and a kitchen domestic for two weeks.

If we consider separately the responses of the 200 senior staff interviews, so-called administrative tasks dominate, with 51 per cent of men and 46 per cent of women mentioning them. We find an officer in charge saying that her job is:

'looking after the care and welfare of residents – medically and socially attending to them. Ordering provisions and cleaning materials, etc. Organizing the staff and their work rotas. Care and maintenance of equipment and generally supervising all aspects.'

In such ways the supervisory role is characterized by administration. Only a very small component of jobs at lower levels involves paperwork. Where this was mentioned by care staff they would generally be referring to the completion of daily reports on residents, frequently required at the end of a shift, or the maintenance of records on residents such as the bathing rota and reports.

The care assistant's job is dominated by physical care for residents, although this task also features as a small part of the senior role. One care assistant remarked that her job entailed:

> 'making beds, bathing, and toileting the patients, taking them to meals and then back, tucking them up in bed and chatting occasionally.'

For both male and female care staff, this constellation of tasks was often mentioned. However, care staff, as already noted, included domestic tasks in their job descriptions. The broad distinction between the care rendered to the resident's person or to his or her personal belongings, and care of the residents' physical environment has been made elsewhere (Imber 1977; Evans *et al.* 1981). Evans and colleagues elaborate this category of care further by considering the qualitative aspects of such physical caring tasks as bathing and toileting of residents which distinguish the care assistant's role from that of the domestic.

It is significant, however, despite these areas of specialism, that staff at all levels are involved in domestic tasks to some degree. The priority given to cleaning and tidying is also reflected in the urgency staff frequently give to the cleaning and tidying of residents themselves. Given the resources of time and energy invested in these activities and the degree to which staff support such tidying operations, we are probably justified in arguing that it is here we must locate the central goal of old people's homes as organizational entities. Let us consider this proposition in the light of patterns of staff activity in these establishments.

The weekly pattern was often constructed around the routine of bed-changing and laundry activities. In some homes this took place throughout the entire establishment on a given day; in other homes different groups were dealt with on a particular weekday. Connected with this domestic purge of the physical environment might be the weekly bath routines for residents. Daily routines were often also constructed around cleaning operations. Residents' rooms would be cleaned during the morning when domestics were on duty and during this operation residents would move elsewhere, often to the public lounges. Even in homes where room cleaning was not a daily practice, the corridors would be polished every morning, with a consequent restriction on resident movement. Public spaces, such as lounges in which residents were concentrated during the daytime, were cleaned during the night. Cleanliness and hygiene thus appeared to assume a central imporance. This is undoubtedly because, in contrast to other facets of care, they are material and visible achievements and can be thought of as indicative of the more private aspects of care provided for residents. An emphasis on displays of care is important. As Patterson found in a study of six homes (1977), care is translated in terms of those routines which display the help given to residents. Staff expected trouble if a lack of care – lack of routine and order – became apparent. In this connection, the cleanliness of residents is made manifest in the bath book which, signed at the end of a weekly bathing cycle, shows that the home contains a full complement of cleaned and inspected residents.

We might ask whether these activities are in themselves meaningful manifestations of care, if they represent deeper and more subtle levels of social care, or whether they are simply tokens of an intention or obligation to care. It cannot be denied that social contact is entailed in the course of undertaking domestic tasks. Research (Oakley 1976) has also pointed to the invisibility of care in the domestic setting and the needs which carers have to translate their concern into material expressions. This need can be no less important to those who staff residential homes. Indeed, it could be argued that because staff are formally contracted to care, the need for staff to demonstrate, formally and materially, that they are meeting their contractual duties is possibly greater than in the informal setting of the home where the parties to a care 'contract' are kin. At another level, it should not surprise us to find an emphasis being placed on housework since many residents report entering care because they can no longer manage to keep themselves or their homes in good order. For residential care to fail to make good such publicly determined deficits in correspondingly public ways could undermine one of the foundations upon which residential legitimacy rests.

One consequence of the priority given to these material aspects of care is the secondary position of social care. For neither day nor night care staff was there any question of putting aside domestic chores in order to enter into social exchange with residents. In one home there was even an open agreement between care staff that only when all staff had finished the domestic and physical care tasks should they – simultaneously – use the remaining few minutes of a shift to talk with residents.

This question of social care in the residential setting is a vexed one, but it is an aspect of residential life with which care-providers have been concerned for some time. Implicit in the term 'care and attention' is the notion that residents should have relief, not only from the physical burdens of coping in the community, but also from the emotional burdens of isolation. Social activity is inevitably entailed in caring at a material and physical level and there is an assumption that social and material care are integrated. Indeed, social contact between staff and resident occurs in the course of engaging in physical care tasks, and with domestic undertakings as well. This is undoubtedly social care, and may explain the low priority given to specific references to social care, but it raises the question of definition. In some studies (Imber 1977), social care focuses upon those arranged activities such as cards, bingo, and outings which punctuate the residential calendar. In other studies, the social aspect of care is located in everyday communication between staff and residents (Raynes, Pratt, and Roses 1979). Evans and colleagues (1981) pursue this line by observing aspects of physical care such as bathing and toileting of old people in an attempt to gauge the extent to which social aspects really are embedded in physical assistance (1981). Were this the case, we might accept that the comprehensiveness implicit in the goal to provide care and attention was achieved. However, Evans and colleagues do not find this to be so, and our observations would support this.

While the weekly bathtime was anticipated by many residents as an occasion when they could legitimately command the attention of one or two members of staff for ten or fifteen minutes, there were often inter-ruptions and demands which diverted staff from giving the undivided attention residents might have appreciated. It was interesting to note, however, that residents would often use these occasions to reminisce or to mention worries and anxieties – in other words, to present themselves as individuals. For staff, it was also an occasion to relax a little with residents as individuals. From an organizational point of view, however, bathtime offered the chance to check residents for bodily ailments and disorders, and to continue the pursuit of cleanliness. At bathtime residents, and frequently staff, related as individuals. But this was an unusual interaction as staff generally addressed whole groups of residents. Even when individuals were being approached, a collective mode of address would be used, implying that the person was actually in a group context. Residents wanting to talk 'too much' presented problems for staff in that this could impede the routine cleaning and tidying tasks. We find, for instance, that those staff who mentioned domestic, physical, or health care tasks amongst their duties were slightly more likely to report resident talk as a problem than was the case for the small number of staff who made some mention of social care as part of their care duties. While there is a suggestion in these findings of different staff orientation to residents we should not construe the social care trend as necessarily a vigorous one, for staff who mentioned social aspects of care also tended to make comments about residents being less than cooperative. To take this tentative trend a little further, social care in the residential setting may simply be a higher level of alertness on the part of staff to the presence of residents as individuals who may have a choice about acquiescing or objecting to certain staff activities. It would remain true to say, however, that staff preoccupations with cleaning and tidying generally eclipse the reality of residents as individuals.

There is little evidence to suggest that social care is a significant part of residential work, although we should note that some staff are more likely to mention this as part of the job than are others. The same is true of health care which also occupies a correspondingly small niche in the care package. Amongst the senior staff, who are more likely to mention social care than care staff, there are some interesting gender differences in seeing social care as part of the job. Twice as many men cited duties concerning the social well-being of their residents as did women. For instance:

'I'm in charge of old people and their welfare – pastoral work, dealing with their problems and physical ailments.'

But, in the case of care assistance, the gender differences are reversed and it is women who are more likely to mention social care. With health care this appears to be the domain of female senior staff (18 per cent) rather than of senior men (6 per cent). One matron perceived her job in the following terms:

> 'I just have to manage everything, the ordering and the drugs, ring-ing the doctor . . . any medical attention.'

The description of daily duties offered by a care assistant shows the extent to which health needs of residents, or sickness care, especially in terms of their medications, are also a concern at this level:

> 'I see to meals and care for residents, serve meals, give out tablets for the next twenty-four hours, prepare meals for the next day, help to put residents to bed and give them supper, go round with the tablets.'

However, the more positive element in health care, rehabilitation in the activities of daily living, is accorded very low priority overall.

The main point to be made is that residential care is rendered primarily in domestic and physical care modes, and that the greatest investment of care staff time is in this facet of care. Such a care edifice is, in turn, organized by senior managers who may offer more social care to residents than do care staff.

Some may argue that this is too harsh and bleak a representation of residential care and that embedded within these material and collec-tive displays of care there rest sentiments and concerns for frail old people who are in need of 'care and attention'. Concern is undoubtedly an influence upon the development of residential care. The notion of welfare arises from an abstract and generalized concern, on the part of society, for those who cannot exist independently. But, how far can we say that residential care goes beyond this idea of collective appease-ment and tackles care at a more immediate and individual level? By considering why staff work in residential care and what they bring to it from outside or from prior experiences, we may further our under-standing of the ways in which care is constructed in practical terms.

Experiences and expectations of staff

Residential care in these hundred homes was administered by a predominantly female workforce; only 7 per cent of all staff listed were male, although at senior level this proportion increased to 16 per cent.

Among the staff sampled for interview, men at both senior and care levels are over-represented; 63 per cent of all male seniors were interviewed as were 35 per cent of all male care staff. Moreover, at senior level a disproportionately high number of officer in charge posts (25 per cent) were held by men – though fourteen of these men undertook their supervisory tasks with wives appointed as assistants or deputies. With very few exceptions, being a senior care officer entails a contract to work a full forty-hour week. However, examination of the data shows that where part-time senior staff were employed these were likely to be women supported, at senior and care level, by other women rather than by men.

These patterns remind us that old people's homes are not entirely isolated from their social contexts. Both the organizational environment, generated by particular policies, and the economic environment, generated by local employment and labour market conditions, have a bearing upon the nature of the care available within a particular home. The staff who are recruited to work in residential settings are, in many respects, products of these contexts and as individuals bring extraneous influences to bear upon the task they undertake and upon the lives of residents. Despite debates as to the relative importance of the personal qualities and experiences of staff and of the training they undergo, the fact is that most care staff approach the task of residential care from a background of common sense caring and experience practised in the domestic setting. For only a small proportion are these prior experiences likely to be modified by formal training.

Prior experiences

The finding that the average age of staff interviewed was 44.3 years – with senior staff averaging six years more than care staff – says something about the life events staff are likely to have experienced. A majority were, or had been, married (68 per cent), single staff being mainly the younger female care staff, and a third of all staff still had children under school-leaving age; for most of the others, families were older. The point hardly needs to be laboured that these staff members were well grounded in child-care and in domestic work, and that these experiences would be transferred to residential work. At the same time it may be less than desirable for care of the elderly to be seen as a variation on a caring theme practised with children. The analogy between frail old people and children is one encountered fairly often in residential care and, while there may be parallels, there are also crucial differences. Although nearly one in five staff, all seniors and almost equally men and women, reported living on site, this is an aspect of residential life which has changed, with staff increasingly moving out to own their own homes. But it is interesting to note that a further third of all staff still lived within a mile of their workplace. These tended to be care staff, suggesting that once senior staff moved off site they ventured further afield. This may be a necessary separation between full-time work and home life as those who had been in the job for several years lived furthest away from the home.

In terms of work experience, staff represented a fairly static group. The manual grading of the care assistant's post, with poor remuneration, possibly combined with a need to find a job close to home, will inevitably restrict these workers' mobility in the job market and lead to the low turnover these hundred homes had experienced with their staffing. Over two-thirds had more than five years' experience, either in the home sampled or in a similar setting. Not surprisingly, senior staff had significantly longer experience than care staff, male seniors having had more time in the job than their female counterparts. At care level as well, men were more likely to have worked for five or more years; two-thirds of male care staff compared to only half of the women were relatively long established. Having children under school-leaving age is one obvious explanation for women's shorter work experience, but this is also linked to age, and male care staff with children were also in this mid-experience bracket. This amounts to most staff having considerable experience in the particular home concerned and the others having worked in similar establishments. The remaining third, however, said that five years earlier they had been engaged in some other activity; the most common was nursing training.

Since over half of these men and women had no formal qualifications relevant to work with old people in the residential setting it is clear that they will draw considerably upon these earlier and non-residential experiences. Staff who had been in the job longest were more likely to have gained some qualification or to be considering this. But perhaps the most disturbing finding is that over a third of senior staff (42 per cent) had no relevant qualification, together with three-quarters (75 per cent) of care staff. These findings are similar to those in the work of Evans *et al.* who reported:

'Whilst it is depressing to find that only half the staff had received any training at all, the content of the in-service courses provided more cause for concern. The courses seemed to largely consist of home nursing with a particular emphasis on first-aid.'(1981: 4: 6)

Rowlings also discusses the extent to which the training of staff in the residential sector has remained a neglected area in comparison with provision for field staff:

'This is in part a consequence of the low status of residential care as a means of helping clients and also contributes to its continuing existence as a residual service.' (1981: 112)

Amongst those who had acquired relevant skills, the most likely form of vocational training at both senior and care levels was nursing (35 per cent and 14 per cent respectively). A rather smaller group of staff, 20 per cent of those with some qualification, reported having a social work training. But only a few of these, twenty-five people, and nearly all seniors, had a residential social work qualification. A few, forty-six, staff members said that they were currently on a training course or were seriously considering one. Where this was the case, training was now more likely to have a social work bias than a nursing one (70 per cent and 13 per cent) so increasing the emphasis on social aspects of caring.

The value of a traditional nursing qualification in a residential setting has been the subject of much debate. In 1978 BASW recognized the contribution it can make, but asserted the need for relevant social work training, possibly to supplement a nursing background which might become more appropriate where residents are more frail (BASW 1978). Indeed, an examination of nursing qualifications in relation to levels of physical impairment in our sample of homes indicated an increase in nursing input which was in direct proportion to raised numbers of frail residents. Thus, in homes with relatively small numbers of physically impaired residents, nursing qualifications account for only 15 per cent of all relevant qualifications. This rises to 30 per cent in those homes with the highest proportions of frail residents (that is 40 per cent or more of residents scoring at least eight on the Crichton Royal assessment of physical impairment).

The fact remains, however, that most staff do not work at caring from a formal training base; rather, they approach the work with sentiments which seem to reflect the generalized rhetoric of the claim that residential care is the provision of care and attention. At the same time, the recognition traditional nursing skills receive seems to legitimize the goals of material and physical orderliness for residents in care and to provide a model around which untrained staff can shape the skills in which they have undoubtedly become proficient on the domestic front.

Staff expectations in the job

While recognizing the complex train of events, motivations, and defaults which lead an individual to a particular job, the constellation of reasons given by staff for starting to work with older people in care is likely to say something about the nature of the images of caring they hold. The models of care discussed at the start of this chapter correspond, to some degree, to the three categories of explanation – altruism, convenience, and continuation of some past experience – derived by factor analysis. The items to which staff were asked to respond are listed below (*Table 4*). Most staff selected two or three of these to describe their reasons for entering residential care.

It is not necessarily cynical to say that we might expect, in such an interview situation, a high proportion of respondents to give 'altruistic' reasons, but we should be cautious in interpreting these socially acceptable responses. The fact that nine out of ten people said they had come to residential work to help people, because of an interest in the elderly, or to do 'nursing', reflects society's ideal of giving care and attention to old people in need, and need not be dismissed simply as padding. Rather, it illuminates both the collectively and personally inspired motivations which lead staff to engage in such caring exchanges.

Table 4   *Three classes of explanations given by staff for first taking a job in an old people's home*

altruistic *reasons*	I wanted to do a job that involved caring for people. I was interested in working with elderly people. I wanted to do (or continue doing) a nursing job. I wanted extra responsibility/challenge.
convenience *reasons*	I was looking for any job. An old people's home was close to my home. The hours and shifts were convenient for me. I was bored (or fed up) with other kinds of work. I was attracted by the pay levels. I wanted a job which provided accommodation.
experience *reasons*	I had a friend/relative who worked with the elderly. I had done voluntary work with elderly people. I had previous experience of relevant work.

Although altruistic explanations predominate, just over half of the staff also recalled a convenience aspect of the work as having been influential (*Table 5*). The convenience of the shifts and of part-time work, as well as being able to work close to home, were given as reasons by many staff. The small number of staff who admitted having been bored with previous jobs and who were prepared to try anything different are included in this convenience category. Finally, a quarter of the staff cited some previous, related experience – perhaps of elderly people, or of old people's homes – as having contributed to their decision.

It would appear that staff, first, justify their involvement in residential care by reference to the rhetoric of altruism – the debt of care due from society as a whole to those of an older generation. Through the altruism associated with the familial caring, in which it is assumed these elderly people have been involved at earlier stages in their lives – probably as parents – their entitlement to a return of care is legitimized, and the ideal of long-term reciprocity is invoked. However, there is a problem in that elderly people in care represent a group for whom this reciprocal ideal has broken down. For all kinds of reasons, those deemed 'responsible' cannot return the debt of care and are obliged to transfer the duty to others. These others must give care on behalf of specifically absent kin and a more generally 'concerned', but also

Table 5   *Types of explanations for working in residential care*

	number	per cent
altruism and convenience	148	37
altruism alone	128	32
altruism and experience	44	11
non-altruistic	41	10
altruism and convenience and experience	38	10
	399	= 100 per cent

absent, society. This legitimizing of residential care, as generalized reciprocity, is reflected in the altruistic explanations staff give. Such, we would argue, is the background against which staff construct ideals, and the framework within which care, in its practical and immediate forms, is delivered. Having set these frameworks, staff then offer more individual and pragmatic reasons for doing the job.

Before examining the pragmatic aspects of staff motivations, let us consider the 10 per cent of people who did not give an altruistic explanation and the larger group who gave only altruistic reasons. For nearly all of the former group the convenience of the work was paramount. A higher proportion of male care staff fall into this group (14 per cent of men compared to 10 per cent of women). They are typically middle-aged workers, married, and unqualified. It is possible that for some people the burden of earning a wage and managing life outside the institution mutes the ideological aspects of caring. We might suggest that in these instances other ideologies, the work ethic for instance, take over. In contrast, quite a large group gave only altruistic reasons. These tended to be women, to be seniors aged forty-five to fifty-four years but with least experience in residential care. A disproportionately high number were divorced, suggesting perhaps that a transfer of caring attentions may be entailed. This group was characterized, where training had been obtained or was being considered, by an orientation towards social work rather than the medical model represented by nursing.

Convenience is valued by over a third who also gave an altruistic reason for doing the job. Here there is no gender differentiation though these staff members are slightly more likely to be in the middle age bracket (twenty-five to fifty-four years) and to be married with family commitments than to be amongst the very youngest or oldest staff. Previous experience or encounter with the world of the residential elderly prompted nearly a quarter of the responses though, again, staff did not often give this explanation on its own. It is interesting that individuals not traditionally associated with caring – men and very young staff – referred to previous experience rather than to convenience as a reason for taking a caring job.

What then might these clusters of motivation mean? First, that caring in the residential world is conceptualized by most staff as being based upon the same principles of altruism as characterize ideals of care, especially between kin. Competing ideologies, such as work, are more likely to typify groups of people who will have received family care – men and younger people – rather than those who have given such care. It might be argued that the ideals of long-term reciprocity held by female care staff are matched in male staff by the more direct reciprocity associated with the market-place. And yet helping people, and helping elderly people needing some nursing care especially, is the explanation which staff voiced most frequently for being in this work. Resident needs for assistance appear to be prominent in staff consciousness. Next, however, we consider what it is that staff themselves might get from doing residential work.

The strains and satisfactions of caring

Much of the recent literature on carers in the community has focused upon the stresses they experience when looking after someone (Finch and Groves 1983). Ungerson (1983) takes this a stage further in discussing the tensions which arise when sexual and pollution taboos are transgressed. The destructive consequences of caring without significant relief from its physical and emotional burdens are also described by Rowlings (1981). The rewards or satisfactions associated with caring are less frequently noted, though Stevenson (1981) discusses the ambiguities entailed in inter-familial dependencies. If we recall the domestic and family idiom, our observation studies show tensions in residential care similar to those which Ungerson cites in family settings surrounding the intimate physical care of residents. Such residential tensions are probably greatest where female staff and male residents are involved, particularly in relation to bathing. The tension occasioned by such events is usually released or transformed by joking, and in any case is often pre-empted by the routine context in which the taboo event is set.

Routine and organization serve to protect staff from many of the stresses associated with caring. Staff work shifts, they get away from the care work, and they have peers with whom they can share anxieties. Guilt and foreboding about death are certainly features of residential life but they are generally suppressed ones. It is the circular timelessness created and imposed by the daily and weekly routines of care which overwhelm the frequent fact of death in residential homes. In other words, organization and routinization make continued caring possible. Given the recent upsurge in attempts to organize relief and support to carers in the community, we might argue that the residential approach is the only feasible one. In other words, it is necessary to routinize the guilt and disorder entailed in caring for frail and elderly people. The scale of care staff tackle both permits and necessitates a distance between the parties. In this respect residential care works, but can we continue to argue that the care given in homes is, or even should be, that provided by 'a caring relative'? The kinship model may be applied in part in the residential setting but we must also concede that this model cannot be maintained consistently. At critical points an organizational model embodying routines will replace kinship models.

Caring is an activity fraught with conflicts and ambiguities, and most staff, as has been shown, have only unsophisticated training to support them in dealing with such problems. Yet reported levels of job satisfaction appeared to be high. Attachment to the caring profession and association with a job which demands altruism are factors which will yield some satisfactions. But, at the practical level, what aspects of the job do staff value and can anything be inferred, about the care given to residents, from the experiences and expectations different groups of staff report in relation to their jobs?

The job of caring in residential settings for old people is conceived here as having three dimensions. First, there is autonomy: the freedom to accomplish necessary tasks using initiative and imagination, being adequately supported and having efforts recognized.

Second, interactions with peers, seniors, and with organizational structures are examined. Third, the contractual conditions in which caring
is undertaken are distinguished. The rankings which emerged on the
sixteen items which made up the job satisfaction index administered
to staff in the interview are shown in *Table 6*. They are grouped within
the three dimensions described above, which in turn were derived by
factor analysis (see Appendix 2).

Table 6 *Job satisfaction scores and rankings for senior and care staff, male and female*

	All	Senior		Care	
		men	*women*	*men*	*women*
job autonomy					
freedom to choose working method	74	74	75	74	73
amount of responsibility given	77	81	80	71	75
attention paid to suggestions	69	71	75	64	65
amount of variety	77	80	81	71	74
recognition for work	69	59	71	74	69
immediate superiors	79	72	78	85	79
way home is managed	75	77	79	71	72
job interactions					
fellow workers	80	79	81	79	79
immediate superiors	79	72	78	85	79
relations between bosses and workers	74	72	74	80	72
job conditions					
physical working conditions	70	71	73	69	67
rate of pay	72	75	76	50	70
hours of work	76	69	74	82	78
job security	80	81	83	71	78
chances of promotion	62	62	67	44	59
overall job satisfaction	75	74	77	71	73
scored to base 100 (7 point score)					

That there is a considerable variation for most items in the level of
satisfaction by men and women and by seniors and care staff suggests
a range of viewpoints, even within the same setting. Overall, female
senior staff appear to find most satisfaction in their jobs, with male care

staff reporting least satisfaction. This may be a reflection of the degree to which residential organization has developed as a response to inputs from women as a numerically stronger work force over a longer period – certainly at care staff level. As a consequence, residential care work – a job to be fitted between family commitments, and perhaps an extension of these – may be less likely to match male ideas about work. Male care staff are less satisfied with job security than are their female counterparts, and the same goes for their satisfaction with pay rates. Other variations suggest that male and female care staff have different orientations to the work. Whereas both groups claim that relations with immediate superiors are highly satisfactory, men appear to be much more satisfied with the way the home is run than are the women, the ranking they assign to this item being more aligned with that given by the senior staff who run the home. This configuration of reported satisfactions for male care staff can be construed as a more traditional and hierarchical orientation. An alternative construction can be placed upon the finding that women, at both care and senior levels, valued interactions with fellow workers as contributing to job satisfaction.

The relationship between job satisfaction and job performance is one which other researchers (Vroom 1964) have explored and which remains elusive. Similarly the connections between satisfaction with work and satisfaction with life as a whole are difficult to gauge, since an enormously variable set of extraneous circumstances must be considered in relation to the complicated job variables already mentioned. It could be hypothesized that a satisfied staff is likely to contribute to, rather than detract from, resident well-being, although there is the counter-argument that a staff group which is organization oriented and which is relatively self-contained and self-centred will work to the detriment, if not the neglect, of the residents. There is clearly an optimum balance between extremes of over-involvement in the staff world and over-involvement in the resident world. Miller and Gwynne (1972), for instance, argue that fewer staff can mean less interference for residents, implying that reduced staff time for residents may have some beneficial aspects.

The organizational dimensions of resident-oriented policies and staff-oriented policies have been developed in the work of King, Raynes, and Tizard (1971). The importance of such analytic work has led to the construction of variables which reflect something of the nature – the culture – of the staff working group. In the course of the detailed studies it emerged that there were sometimes groupings of staff which appeared to be particularly cohesive and exclusive of residents. There were other instances where staff interacted only minimally with each other, directing their attentions and efforts towards the residents. Clearly, levels of cohesion and dispersal of the staff group will vary within a particular home from time to time – perhaps from shift to shift depending upon staff personalities and friendships. But are there any more durable factors, controllable at the level of organization, which have a bearing upon the nature of staff groupings and, most importantly, upon resident lifestyle and well-being?

A range of organizational factors contributes to the shape which a particular staff complement may assume. The ratio of staff hours to resident numbers is one of these, and the allocations of staff to each of the categories already enumerated in *Figure 3* is another. In addition, there is a limited range of strategies an employing authority can adopt to arrive at a given establishment of staff and at a particular pattern of care delivery. The main pivots of such strategies are, first, the employment of more or less part-time staff, and second, the fixing of shifts. Certain permutations of all these factors and strategies will lead to staffing arrangements which are more or less fragmented in terms of personnel and in terms of shift periods. It is arguable that different levels of fragmentation may have consequences for the staff team and for staff working life and may also, directly or indirectly, impinge upon resident groupings and their well-being in the residential setting. A hypothesis may be set up that greater fragmentation of the workforce will be confusing for both residents and staff and will make the environment too busy. On the other hand there is the counter hypothesis that such arrangements will enrich the milieu by enlarging the potential social contacts for both groups concerned.

Across the hundred homes, taking supervisory, care, and domestic hours into account, some two and a quarter hours of staff time are available to each resident each day (0.44 senior hours, 1.3 care staff hours, and 0.5 domestic hours per resident, per day). Staff job satisfaction is lowest in those twenty-two homes where the average time available from seniors, care staff, and domestics to care for each resident is below the average. In particular, staff in these homes had lower job autonomy scores. Working methods and variety in the work are likely to be restricted where time allows for only the essentials to be tackled. The finding that staff-oriented policies are strongest in these same homes with lowest resources lends support to the idea that formalization is necessary in order for tasks to be completed. Flexibility for staff, and for residents, may consequently have to be dispensed with in such circumstances. It has been suggested (e.g. in Raynes, Pratt, and Roses 1979: 37) that lowered staff morale may follow upon formalization and our findings on lowered job autonomy support this proposition.

The second finding concerning overall staffing strategies is that enhanced staff job satisfaction scores are associated with higher numbers of part-time staff and a high proportion of care hours being undertaken by part-timers. These findings together suggest, not surprisingly, that staff appreciate more resources which give them greater scope and variety in their jobs, and also that the demands of the care task may better be controlled and contained by part-time strategies which give staff more frequent respite and recovery times. Additionally staff score highly on the interaction dimension of job satisfaction where part-time contracts are typical. The other point to be made here is that raised care staff satisfaction levels appear to be associated with increases in domestic staffing rather than with increases in senior input. It is interesting that senior staff, who often stand in for absent care, domestic, or kitchen staff, may be more valued for their contributions on these fronts than for any supervisory role they may enact.

There is some evidence to show that job satisfaction may be influenced by certain staffing strategies. There is only a little evidence, however, to suggest, very tentatively, how residents' lives may be touched by these constellations of staffing arrangements. First, we find that homes with more plentiful staffing resources and with arrangements which tend towards the part-time rather than the full-time, have more resident-oriented policies and more agreement between staff and residents on what constitute ideal environmental features.

The ethos in residential homes is towards homogeneity and congruence and away from conflicts, but it is clear that the two domains of staff and residents differ in many respects. We should ask whether high levels of reported agreement between staff and resident groups in particular homes are satisfying for residents. Only in the thirteen homes characterized by reduced staff hours and high numbers of part-time staff is there any suggestion that residents' lives are affected by these kinds of arrangements. In these homes resident satisfaction is reduced. Interestingly though, within those homes where staff satisfaction levels are lowest, resident satisfaction is raised. Here we might cautiously argue that we can see just the hint of a difference between resident and staff interests. For the other homes, however, there is no discernible pattern of differences between staff and resident groups.

Other researchers have suggested that residents' well-being may be enhanced where they are relatively free from staff 'interference' (Lipman and Slater 1977a). Our evidence is not strong enough to confirm such claims, but in this chapter we have attempted to show that the staff world, while depending upon the resident world for its existence is, in many respects, independent of that resident world. At the same time, the separate work world of staff as an organized labour force is not consistently and overtly recognized. Rather, the altruistic model of caring in the kinship mode is to the fore – without justification it can be argued – for the care rendered to residents is predominantly physical care. Social care is not a significant component of the package and it is probably true to say that the satisfactions staff get from caring are a consequence of their capacity to organize and control the demands made upon them in ways which are not typical of family and community settings.

Although the organizational model is one which underpins residential caring, it is often obscured behind images and ideals of kinship reciprocities and exchange. It is curious then that the domestic side of residential care does not emerge as a stronger and more distinct entity. Rather, it appears that domestic images and realities – insofar as they exist in residential settings – are converted into organizational units with which staff can work.

One consequence of these transformations is that residential care is created by organizational forces and by the staff group rather than by the resident group or 'domestic' influences. The nature of the care which emerges is not, then, of the relatively embedded, partially visible kind we traditionally associate with family caring. Residential care becomes a highly visible and public affair through which staff justify themselves in interaction with the private individuals for whom the residential world is home.

CHAPTER 5

The physical world

Our understanding of the lives of both residents and staff in old people's homes would be incomplete if it was not set in context. The environment therefore becomes a crucial factor in our analysis and in this chapter we focus on the impact of built form, on the lives of those who use residential buildings, and on their relationship with the wider community. Consideration of the social environment, although obviously related, forms the essential material of the next chapter.

The physical environment can be viewed from both functional and symbolic perspectives. Although it appears to many that the success of a building lies in whether or not it fulfils the purpose for which it was designed and meets the needs of those who use it, built form can also embody and reinforce a particular ideology. For local authority architects involved in the design or conversion of a residential home for elderly people the brief, as reflected in official guidance, demands a compromise between domestic and institutional architecture that accommodates the needs of both residents and staff. Yet the fact that many of the purpose-built homes in the National Consumer Study still conveyed an institutional image suggests that architects have failed to reach such a reconciliation. This raises the important questions: Has the residential home been designed with the needs of the residents or the staff in mind? Can a building which must house as many as forty residents ever be truly 'domestic' in character?

Residential homes in perspective

Although much of what is discussed in this chapter focuses upon the importance of internal spatial arrangements in homes, the external appearance of buildings can also make an important statement to the outside world. To reiterate the quote from the 1973 Building Note:

> 'The style of the homes for elderly people, both externally and internally, should be domestic as befits function, and an institutional appearance is to be avoided.' (DHSS and Welsh Office 1973: 5)

How we read buildings can depend on a number of interesting concepts: imageability – how features such as size and design make the building stand out from its surroundings; visibility – the importance of the building in terms of its use; movement – what kinds of activities occur near the building; and finally, the cultural significance of the building within the wider community (Appleyard 1969, 1970).

The imageability of the old people's home is best understood by a consideration of the overall shape of the building, defined by an examination of vertical height and horizontal ground plan. Over the years a recognition of the mobility needs of the frail elderly has resulted in homes with fewer storeys, but with larger and more complex floor plans. This has been especially true of most recent purpose-built group unit homes. Of the hundred homes studied, half of those opened before 1960 had three storeys whereas 70 per cent of homes provided during the 1970s were on one or two floors. A majority of the twenty-three group or semi-group living homes in the study built during the 1960s and 1970s had two floors. By combining height with ground plan we can arrive at the simple typology of home-type given in *Figure 4*. This distinguishes between simple, semi-complex, and complex building forms, and shows that as ground plans have become more complex, vertical simplicity has become more evident. Such a typology can be further refined by the addition of size of home, based on the number of resident places available. The outcome shows that small (forty places and less) and simple homes are more typical of those opened prior to 1960 whereas in more recent years larger and more complex homes have been provided for greater numbers of residents.

Such a typology suggests that the local authority residential home may have become more rather than less visible again in the community. However, the type of image that is projected may also depend on location.

> 'We couldn't believe they were going to build so close. There's a lack of privacy; they said they'd put thick net curtains but even with the curtains you can see people peering out at you. They also cut down loads of trees; I call it vandalism, they shouldn't be allowed to. But of course it's council, so what could we do?'

and

> 'Well, we were totally overlooked so we complained. The architect had to alter the windows upstairs.'

The feelings expressed by these home-owners also convey something of the nature of institutions that sets them apart, symbolically and functionally, from the 'normal' environment (Canter and Canter 1979; Harvey 1970). The building may be associated with a lack of movement, residents seldom being seen out in the community or in the grounds of the home except when sitting out on a sunny day. And such movement as there is may reinforce the public stereotype of ageing and its association with disablement – the coming and going of ambulances and minibuses or the sight of old people in wheelchairs or moving slowly with zimmer frames. In terms of visibility and cultural significance the local authority home may be experienced, at worst, as invisible; by the majority with indifference; and at best, from a paternalistic or philanthropic standpoint. Such perceptions reflect the status of both the frail elderly and the publicly owned buildings in which they live. In contrast with the domestic home, these buildings fail to convey any sense of personal ownership, of territoriality, or of individual influence over external appearance. These are all features which suggest that the occupants are distanced from their environments. To the community at large, residential homes reinforce a view which conveys an impression that residents are a homogeneous group of 'old people' lacking personal identity or individuality.

Figure 4 A rudimentary typology of 100 homes
An attempt was made to classify the 100 homes into types: three
characteristics were taken into consideration, horizontal plan (simplicity or
complexity), vertical section (number of floors), and size of home (number
of residents).

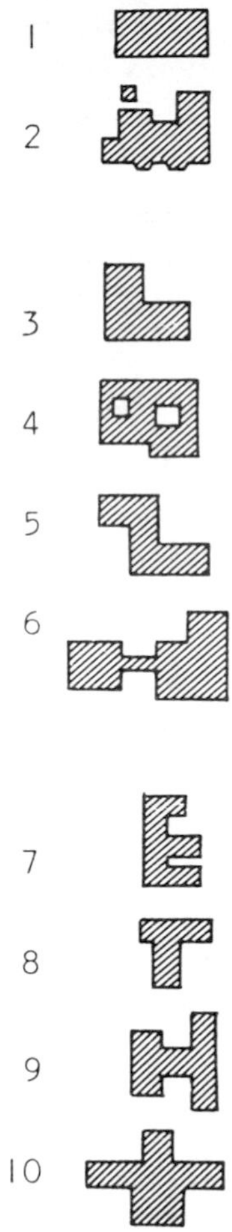

Simple – characterized by a single block having no
extensions or wings and having a unitary plan   1

1 rectangular
2 irregular   2

Semi-complex – consisting of two or more blocks,
joined, with circuit-through routes   3

3 L -shaped
4 around court(s)
5 L -shaped   4
6 distinct blocks linked by passage or bridge

                                                                 5

                                                                 6

Complex – characterized by an arrangement of
adjoining blocks or wings which form cul-de-sacs   7

7   E -shaped
8   T -shaped   8
9   H -shaped
10 + -shaped

                                                                 9

                                                                 10

type A: small and simple   16 homes
type B: medium and semi-complex   47 homes
type C: large and complex   35 homes

Figure 4 contd.

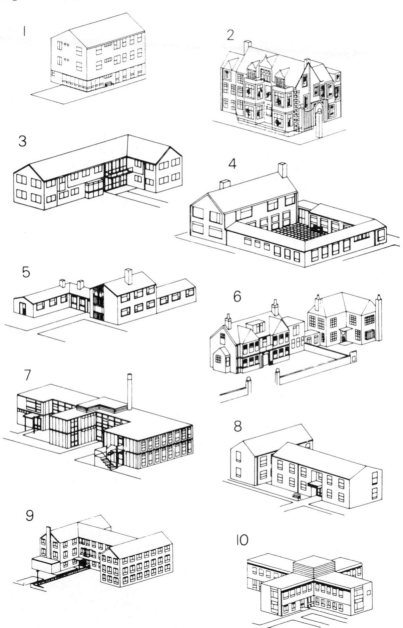

Internal spatial arrangements

It is common to describe the internal spatial arrangements of domestic buildings in terms of public and private space (Rapoport 1982; Lawrence 1982) and our detailed observations within four homes confirmed the importance of these divisions within the residential setting. Public space includes lounges, dining-rooms, halls, and circulation spaces. Private spaces consist of bedrooms, bathrooms, and WCs. It is true that in public spaces such as lounges, certain strategies may be employed by residents to ensure a degree of privacy, and the private spaces, such as bedrooms and bathrooms, can become relatively public. However, the public/private distinctions of space – which follow traditional patterns and expectations of congregation and segregation – did persist in most homes.

Although the public and private spatial distinction could be applied to all residential homes, the distribution, and hence the integration of such areas varied with the size, complexity, and age of the building. An examination of the amount and variety of space provided for each resident shows that since the 1970s there has been a considerable increase in the amount of private space provided, notably through private single bedrooms. But this has not been at the expense of public space, which has also increased, though less dramatically. An example of an integrated spatial arrangement can best be seen in the group living model where bedroom and lounge/dining areas are intermixed, whereas adapted property, with a modern extension accommodating a bedroom wing, may be said to be segregated insofar as the public and private spaces are quite separate (*Figures 5* and *6*). Several authors have commented on the importance of internal scale in facilitating resident behaviour. Lawton (1970) comments that activities of daily living are more easily maintained if toilets, bathrooms, and dining facilities are situated close to sitting areas and Rosow has suggested that the proximity of residents' rooms is an important determinant in friendship formation (1967). However, it can be shown that the spatial proximity and functional centrality of areas within the building are only one influence on social integration.

Figure 5 Very integrated homes – where bedrooms, bathrooms, and WCs are sited close to lounges and dining areas.*

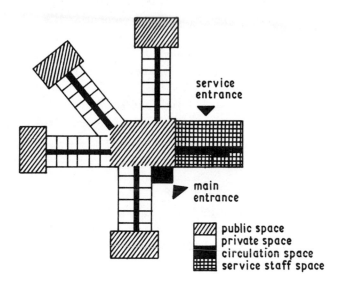

Figure 6 Very separate homes – where clusters of lounges often adjacent to the dining-room are some distance from the bedroom/bath block.*

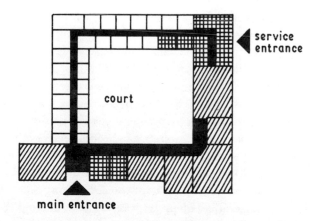

Note. The floorplans used throughout the text are symbolic representations of ground-floor plans only – derived from homes in the study.

Design for living

While it is not our intention to argue for architectural determinism, the characteristics of the physical environment and the absence or presence of certain facilities are, nevertheless, important with respect to potential resident/staff behaviour. Opportunities for resident autonomy and self-determination may be enhanced by aspects of design, even where these may be mediated through the actions of staff. What then are the essential design features of the residential environment, given that the average home in the study accommodated about forty residents?

Standards

At the time of this study the official guidance for standards of physical provision within statutory old people's homes was contained in the 1973 Building Note: Residential Accommodation for Elderly People. *Table 7* indicates official standards and the percentage of homes, from the study, which met these requirements.

Eleven homes in the study met all these requirements; thirty-one homes met four out of the five requirements. Yet these figures mask a wide variation between homes, which relates to the date when the home was opened, to its original function, and to the size and design of the building. Such differences are not apparent in the distributions of public and private space. In the public areas, lounges and dining-rooms serve as the main arena for residents' activities during the day. An examination of the 427 lounges in the 100 homes revealed that, over time, the number of lounges in homes had increased, yet this investment had not occurred at the expense of overall sitting space or bedroom space. This trend reflects the preponderance of large sitting-rooms in those converted homes which were brought into service in the 1950s; this differs from the later move to purpose-built homes which incorporated more small lounges. An increase in the variety of lounges, both in number and décor, permits resident choice of sitting area, although organizational imperatives often suppress decision-making. Resident choice of lounge may also be restricted due to the amount of space provided per resident, the shape of rooms, and the arrangement of

Table 7   *Number of homes meeting space requirements*

	local authority Building Note recommendation	percentage of homes meeting recommendation
sitting space	3.7 m^2 per resident	56
single bedroom	10.0 m^2 per resident	47
double bedroom	15.5 m^2 per resident	50
bathrooms	1 per 15 residents	80
WCs	1 per 4 residents	94
		N = 100

chairs. Moreover, in many lounges, only enough chairs for residents, and perhaps for the occasional day-attender, were provided. Thus social activities such as visiting were often undertaken in difficult circumstances. Additional sitting areas were sometimes located in hallways or on circulation routes.

Seventy-four homes had one main dining-room and the remainder included several smaller dining–sitting areas. In fifty-four of the hundred homes studied, the dining-room could be said to form a 'focal' point in the home. This was possibly because, in line with Building Note recommendations, most dining-rooms were adjacent to kitchens and, as mealtimes were the main daily activity for residents and staff alike, the hub of home life commonly revolved around the dining-room. In this sense dining-rooms bridged resident and staff domains and were also often busy thoroughfares.

The central pull of these public spaces was often reinforced by the multiple use of both lounges and dining-rooms. This is also recommended in the Building Note and both areas were used not only for group gatherings such as social functions and religious services but also for more personal activities such as hairdressing and chiropody. If these activities were not forced into the public arena then they were commonly undertaken in 'special' rooms. A minority of homes, notably the more recent purpose-built homes, had a range of additional rooms to meet these special needs. Only medical rooms and staff rooms were more generally provided (*Table 8*).

Yet the allocation of particular rooms for special purposes may also result in potentially private and informal activities taking place in formal, public, and semi-public spaces – for instance, visits with the

Table 8 *Homes with separate facilities for special purposes*

facility	no. of homes
medical/clinic/doctor's room	78
staff/office/common room	76
laundry/washing/ironing room	49
visitors' room/overnight visitor's room	38
sewing room	34
residents' tea-making/snack-making/kitchenette	25
chiropody/hairdressing room	24
storage room, e.g. linen/stock-room/cleaners' room	15
residents' laundry/washing room	15
sick room	13
residents' recreation room for hobbies/handicrafts plus bar	13
staff duty/night duty room	8
residents' shop	6

doctor that could be carried out in a resident's bedroom being undertaken in the medical room. Barrett argues that the number of so-called 'institutional rooms', for example visitors' rooms, should be kept as low as possible, whereas 'non-institutional rooms', for example kitchenettes, should be encouraged (1976). However, in practice, the use made of all special rooms in the hundred homes was found to be contingent upon organization routines, and in some cases they were under-utilized, degenerating into extra storage space.

We have argued that the character of the physical environment derives from the integration or segregation of public and private space in the home. In a similar way the character of private space rests upon the balance of single to multiple occupancy bedrooms. For instance, where there is a concentration of residents in rooms for three people, there tends to be a sharper division between public and private areas, and the building is likely to be simple rather than complex in design.

Multiple occupancy bedrooms occur typically in homes opened during the 1950s and 1960s. Those with a high proportion of treble rooms were most likely to be adapted homes, whereas high proportions of double bedrooms are common in adapted homes with modern extensions and in the large purpose-built homes of the 1960s. Homes with a high proportion of single bedrooms also tended to be large, with more than fifty residents, but had usually been constructed in the 1970s and were often of the group unit design. To a certain extent such trends reflect ministerial guidance which since 1954 has recommended single bedrooms (Barrett 1976), and supports the findings of Knapp that the number of single rooms and occupancy is due to original function, age, and size of home (1977).

Bedroom size also varied with the type and age of the home. Double rooms averaged 19.8 square metres in adapted homes, 16.1 square metres in purpose-built homes, and 14.7 square metres in purpose-built group unit homes. The size of a double room often dictates whether it is possible to arrange furniture in such a way that the room contains distinct territories. While a double or treble room may be suitable as a bedsitting room, this potential was only rarely realized. In many cases the need for access space near the door often restricted the positioning of beds and chests of drawers. Moreover it may prove difficult to install individual easy chairs and other pieces of furniture, hence the sharing of space by two or three comparative strangers may be constructed in terms of a safe neutrality rather than as expressions of individuality.

Fifty-three per cent of single bedrooms fell short of the recommended 10 square metres. However, in terms of resident lifestyle, the mere fact of having a room of one's own may be more important than its size (Norman 1984) and in more than two-thirds of the homes it appeared that single rooms had the potential for use as bedsitting rooms. They were equipped not only with an easy chair, but also with an electric power socket, so that residents could watch their own television or boil a kettle in their room. Nevertheless, only half of all the residents in the hundred homes had single bedrooms.[1]

In contrast, the provision of bathrooms and WCs throughout the hundred homes was more likely to meet the required standards. This reinforces the emphasis placed on physical care. The range of bath type provided varied across the homes. All homes had at least one ordinary full-length bath, usually equipped with some form of grab-bar or grip to support residents as they got in or out of the bath. Other types of bath commonly found were medibaths and baths with ambulifts. Few homes had more than one of these; most had one or the other. Both types of bath require a degree of staff assistance that restricts the frequency with which they can be used, and yet they were said by staff to be of great assistance in bathing immobile or disabled residents. These quite complex pieces of machinery were found across the range of homes and in some they had been installed through staff fund-raising efforts in order to replace an ordinary bath. Such efforts had been initiated primarily to assist the work routines of staff rather than to enhance the lives of residents.

Separate shower rooms were found in only nineteen homes, although most homes had shower attachments in bathrooms, some of which were attached to and used in conjunction with the medibaths. Staff commented that, in the main, residents did not like using the showers as they were unused to them and preferred a bath:

> 'There is no real use for showers because residents prefer to bathe. Occasionally showers are used on the men, but most residents are more secure in a bath and would be very distressed to have water sprayed on them.'

This is just one instance where the popular view may pre-empt resident choice.

All but six homes had enough WCs to meet the Building Note recommendations of one WC to every four residents. However, of more importance is the siting and distribution of WCs (Barrett 1976). One in ten officers in charge felt that there were not enough well-positioned WCs and that the siting of some were offensively prominent. These WCs tended to be the ones which served daytime public areas in homes where there was a sharp division between public and private areas. In such cases a few WCs had to serve the majority of residents who remained in the public areas for most of the day.

With regard to the segregation of WCs for men and women, residents, especially women, tended to say that they preferred separate facilities, and this was particularly true in the larger homes. Just over a quarter of the homes made no provision for separate facilities, whereas in thirty-one homes all WCs were either for men or for women. In the remaining homes it was common to have segregated facilities near to public areas, with those in more private areas of the home being undesignated. Inevitably, given the greater number of women in residential homes, segregated facilities near dining-rooms or lounges will become congested, a telling example of the failure of designers to respond to the special characteristics and needs of their consumers.

In addition to providing a living environment for residents, homes must also provide a suitable working environment for staff. For this reason, staff rooms, duty rooms, kitchens, laundries, and on-site staff accommodation have to be provided and this results in an increase in overall home size. All of the homes in the study had a central kitchen, usually equipped to commercial standards. Here the main meals were prepared for residents and in some cases the catering was undertaken for local meals-on-wheels delivery. A separate area was also allocated for laundry, which in most cases consisted of residents' personal washing, with heavier laundry being sent out. In some older establishments washing took place in an adapted sluice room whereas in the more modern buildings a well-equipped laundry was provided.

On-site accommodation for senior staff, either in the form of a staff house or flat, was provided within or adjacent to all of the hundred homes. Most of this accommodation was occupied by residential staff, and those few flats that were not utilized by residential staff either accommodated other social services staff or had been turned into a group unit for the more active residents. Comments concerning on-site accommodation by staff centred on a lack of privacy, poor sound-proofing, and the need for separate entrances to flats. Such short-comings, coupled with the changing status of residential work and a desire by staff to separate their working and private lives, have contributed to the accelerating trend among senior staff to live away from the home.

While on-site accommodation was generous, other staff facilities were often lacking. Only half the homes had staff rooms, and yet this was usually the only place where staff could relax. Moreover, the rooms provided were often too small to accommodate all the staff at one time, resulting in domestic and care staff using the room at different times. In the main, staff rooms were used for coffee and meal breaks, and as cloakrooms. A third of the homes also had some kind of duty room with a kitchen and bedroom and in some cases a bathroom. Duty rooms were used by senior staff on call or by care staff on night duty. Apart from these facilities all homes had a main office. This was used exclusively by senior staff and/or administrative staff and it was often sited near to the main entrance of the home.

The integration or segregation of staff and resident facilities within institutional settings has been the subject of much discussion, and authors like Barrett (1976) and Lipman and Slater (1977a) argue that, by increasing the physical distance between staff and residents, surveillance and other dependency-inducing practices may be reduced, while interactions between residents may increase.

These detailed characteristics of the physical environment reflect changes in both the design of, and policy concerning, residential homes for old people over several decades. Improvements in the standards of physical provision, especially the increase in the number of single bedrooms, have resulted in a change in the overall size and appearance of the residential home. However, current provision, as we have seen, is far from uniform and such variation in the physical fabric of the homes may have important implications for the lives of residents and staff. In our discussion so far we have contrasted the rhetoric of residential care with what we know of the domestic lives of older people in the community; we have considered the circumstances and characteristics of elderly residents and the working lives of staff; and we have begun to understand something of the inherent conflicts in care settings. In the next section we explore the relationship between the physical environment and resident and staff behaviour by examining a number of facets of residential life which further highlight these contradictions. Privacy, autonomy, negotiability, safety, and community integration are simple labels for complex concepts which have been elaborated elsewhere (Ittelson *et al.* 1974). Here we consider them in relation to everyday experiences of residential life.

Privacy

The analogy of the domestic home as compared with residential care reveals the different levels of privacy associated with each setting. Given the experience of old people within their own homes, the maintenance of privacy, as defined within our culture, may have an important influence on resident well-being. We can define various levels of privacy ranging from the complete separation of solitude to the anonymity of being within a group and yet apart from it (Westin 1967). While certain kinds of privacy obviously do not pertain within domestic settings, in a residential home different modes of privacy become more important, thus illustrating the dissimilarity between the two environments.

Within this context, solitude implies that the individual can be separate from the group and unobserved by others. This entails seclusion within a personal space. Yet we have noted that only half of all the residents in the hundred homes had a bedroom of their own. The others shared, mainly with one or two others, but in a few cases with as many as seven. Opportunities for solitude may, therefore, be limited and even those with a room of their own may be prevented from experiencing privacy. Only eight of the homes had bedrooms that were lockable, and in only two were residents allowed to lock their rooms from the inside. We can argue that space which is not defensible undermines the sense of ownership which residents may wish to attach to their rooms; without such control this private space becomes common territory.

Within the broad concept of privacy, intimacy entails the needs of people who are close, such as family or friends, to get together in seclusion to talk, share activities, express their sexuality, or just be together. These are important aspects of life which do not translate well to institutional settings. The quality of visiting may be affected by the kind of privacy available for such meetings. While nearly half of the residents used their own rooms for such visits, many were forced to use public spaces such as lounges and hallways. Thirty-eight of the homes in the study had a visitors' room but in many cases these rooms were underused, being rather formal places which deterred intimate conversation.

In contrast to the desire to be with chosen others, the need to be anonymous in a public setting represents a facet of personal privacy. Within our own homes the living-room or sitting-room becomes public space in that people from outside are admitted. However, it is not usually a place in which we expect to feel anonymous. Yet, in the lounge of an old people's home, anonymity may take on a new meaning. The sedentary and passive nature of residential life often provokes comment from practitioners, especially on the arrangement of chairs in lounges and the tendency for residents to occupy particular chairs. Unlike the resident's bedroom, the chair in the lounge may become defensible space, and it is common to see chairs adorned with blankets and cushions, defended by the owner's zimmer frame.

In most of the lounges in the hundred homes, chairs were positioned around the walls or in rows, rather than in arrangements thought to be conducive to social interaction. Whether chair arrangements should be changed in order to encourage interaction or whether residents prefer the present arrangement has been the subject of much debate (Lipman 1967b). In the present study residents and staff voiced differences: staff preferred the arrangement which appears less institutional but residents preferred chairs placed around the walls or in rows facing the television set. It can be argued that, at a purely practical level, this latter choice supports the need to have spacious access to and from lounges for elderly people who may need to use walking aids. However, it also has to be acknowledged that this arrangement allows residents to avoid prolonged social interaction and to withdraw to relative anonymity. There is, after all, no reason why residents – generally strangers to each other – should wish to engage in continuous interaction, especially when they may be sitting in the same seats for up to eight hours a day. If this period were not so long then interaction might be more acceptable. The 'backs to the wall' strategy may be construed as a retreat position, and the somewhat uninterested focusing upon the television as a further strategy for avoiding eye contact with other residents.

Autonomy

The degree to which residents determine their own lifestyle within the residential home will vary with individual personality and through the constraints placed upon people by the organizational style of the home. The physical environment may be thought of as secondary, although it is possible to identify situations where the physical environment either facilitates or hinders resident autonomy. Moreover, we can argue that an institutional environment which is resource-rich has the potential for enhancing resident autonomy through environmental control. In this respect the importance of having a single bedroom is once again brought into focus. While we have noted that the single bedroom offers the resident the potential for privacy, it also offers the potential for an expression of self-identity in the form of personal territory or as a power base from which the resident may engage in some form of exchange relationship with staff. This relationship contains a number of factors, not least the expectations of residents and staff concerning the functions of care.

The concept of bedsitting room was more generally understood by residents who had a single room rather than a shared room, and there was, not surprisingly, a significant association between residents who brought to the home items such as televisions, radios, and furniture and their labelling of rooms as bedsitters, thus confirming the relationship between personalization and the more varied use of bedroom space. Personalization was most common in single rooms that were slightly larger than the average 10 square metres. Many single rooms revealed a remarkable design ingenuity in that the basic trappings of daily life were represented within a small space. At the same time the token nature of such efforts was obvious, given the restrictions posed by fitted furniture – most frequently a washbasin and a wardrobe.

Control of the immediate environment was also something to which residents attached considerable importance. In the visual game, over two-thirds of respondents signalled the importance of the following items: openable windows, easily opened doors, storage space, good sound insulation between rooms, and a power point in the bedroom. In seventy-eight of the homes residents were said by staff to be able to open their bedroom windows. In sixty-eight homes all rooms had at least one electric socket and in sixty-four homes residents could regulate the heater in their rooms. Yet in only a third of homes could residents control all three of these environmental features. In only half of the homes were residents provided with somewhere in their bedrooms to lock away small private possessions, a problem remarked upon by a third of the residents. Thus scope for personal control was very basic, and available to only a minority of residents.

While personal autonomy for residents within an institutional setting is constrained by the existing operational policy, the availability of certain physical resources may encourage, or at least underpin, a more independent lifestyle. Yet relatively few homes had facilities for residents to make a cup of tea or coffee, a shop within the home, or an activities room (see *Table 8*). All these amenities may enable some residents to maintain everyday domestic activities or encourage them to take up new hobbies.

Negotiability

Within the context of negotiating the home environment, three themes are particularly important: rights of access, orientation, and ease of mobility. Each of these can significantly influence resident behaviour.

Rights of access

Within homes in the community, most household members have rights of access to all rooms in their house or flat. Such rights may of course be modified. For example, children may have limited access to their parents' bedroom or a front room may be under-utilized except when visitors call. These are modifications which develop through traditional custom and practice and they reflect a separation of public and private spaces in domestic settings; they do not reflect a separation of living and working spaces for two distinct groups within the same setting. Yet within the old people's home there are several areas to which residents do not have free access – for example service areas such as kitchens, laundries, boiler rooms, garages, as well as staff living-in accommodation, night duty rooms, and staff common rooms. Residents would not generally expect total access, given the traditions and explicit rules prevailing in institutional settings. However, such exclusions will distance residents from tasks which concern basic activities such as providing and preparing food, washing clothing, and arranging for heating. In an environment where a high percentage of residents are women, the separation from domestic activities is particularly problematic, and it has been only in recent years that homes have given residents facilities for making tea or coffee when they wish, an amenity which is still not universal.

In some ways, rights of access within the residential homes are also defined by circulation spaces – routeways through the building. Circulation spaces have both connecting and separating functions; they enable people to move between places and they also mark the boundaries of spaces. While these spaces tend to have a public rather than a private character, this can change according to the kind of areas served by the route. In private spaces such as bedroom areas, circulation space should buffer as well as link the public spaces. It is also important that these circulation spaces maintain a semi-private character so as to support rather than erode the private areas. In some group-living design homes, where public and private areas are integrated, main circulation routes pass through private areas, thus reducing privacy but increasing rights of access. To counteract this problem, some architects have created a form of buffer by placing bedroom doors in recesses off the main corridors.

Staff have rights of access to all circulation routes as a consequence of their duty to care for and watch over residents. Residents, however, behaved as if there were a policy of restricted access. They were rarely to be found on routes other than those which linked the particular private and public spaces they were accustomed to use. Occasionally the fitter – and most typically male – residents used the main routes for exercise and for chatting.

Orientation

Familiarity with a building often means that it is comprehensible; we know what to expect from it in terms of limitations and possibilities. Yet in residential homes there has been a trend towards large and more complex buildings which may affect orientation. It has been suggested that ambiguity and complexity may be necessary if we are to be engaged by and participate in a particular environment (Rapoport and Kantor 1967). On the other hand, it has also been noted that difficulty in forming a mental picture of an organization in spatial terms may lead to the individual's greater reliance upon those who work in the organization – in other words to greater dependency, if not total passivity (Canter and Canter 1979). The large and complex building, instead of offering a variety of settings, may limit activity and reinforce feelings of disorientation and bewilderment not typical of smaller adapted homes. The use of appropriate signs to identify parts of the building was not common in the homes studied and systematically maintained colour coding was extremely rare, although toilets and resident bedrooms were often identified in some way.

Ease of mobility

It was noted earlier that many residents suffer mobility problems and have to negotiate their environment using a walking aid or a wheelchair. Ease of mobility is therefore an important feature of resident autonomy and here the prosthetic nature of the physical environment becomes very important. At the very broad level of spatial arrangements, the degree of integration between public and private spaces is fundamental to mobility. Where sitting and dining areas are quite separate from bedroom areas, the old person needs considerable independent mobility to make use of both settings unaided. Long corridors linked by steps or ramps represented serious physical obstacles to frail, elderly residents, and provided a partial explanation for the concentrations of residents in public spaces during the daytime.

The problem of the distance between facilities is highlighted in relation to the provision of WCs which must be provided in places accessible from both public and private spaces. Yet in large, traditionally organized homes they tend to serve one or other zone. The public and communal nature of residential life means that those in bedroom areas are under-utilized during the day; indeed they will not even be needed at night as residents habitually use commodes. The most successful solution to this problem was found either in group unit homes, where public and private spaces were adjacent, or in those few homes which had WCs distributed along wings between bedrooms but within easy reach of public areas. In this way the public/private boundary is maintained together with some privacy for residents.

Given that supervised bathing arrangements are usual in residential homes, neither the number of baths available nor the siting of bathrooms was seen as particularly problematic by staff except in some older adapted properties. Residents usually have a bath once a week, in some cases at a set time and day, and long trips to the bathroom can be speeded up in a wheelchair if necessary. However, the size of the bathroom and the location of the bath can become a problem and over a third of staff interviewed commented on limited bathroom space. Yet while centrally placed baths in standard sized bathrooms were seen to lead to congestion, baths positioned against walls caused staff problems when lifting residents.

Nevertheless, distances between facilities can hinder negotiations for residents, as does the amount of space provided in enclosed areas. In many homes there was not enough space within WCs for those who used either wheelchairs or walking aids or those who needed assistance, and the space provided in dining-rooms, especially in group living homes, could also be problematic for those with mobility problems. In some cases the least mobile residents had to be seated first as staff could not get wheelchairs between tables once the residents sat down. As a result, forty-one officers-in-charge commented that the dining-rooms were too small and one solution to the problem was the introduction of two mealtime sittings. Staff commented that the design of the building can directly affect behaviour, home routines, and consequently resident lifestyle:

> 'It becomes cramped with wheelchair users and this means that wheelchair residents have to be put in convenient places, they can't go anywhere they want.'

Ease of mobility within different parts of the building can obviously be assisted by the availability of prosthetic aids to daily living. Lifts, grab-bars, hand-rails, and ramps can all make the environment more accessible to a frail or disabled older person, yet the availability of such devices varied widely. Four out of five homes had rails and handgrips in all WCs; only two of the sampled homes had no rails in any toilets. Yet, while 90 per cent of the homes had handrails along the corridors, nearly one in five homes had corridors that were interrupted by steps – a particular feature of older adapted properties and a definite hindrance to mobility. Twenty-nine homes had rooms that were difficult to reach or inaccessible for residents, either because of the distance to the room or because of steps or stairs in corridors. In a further eight, access to the grounds was difficult for residents unaided by staff due to steps and slopes or the need to negotiate heavy doors.

Eighty of the homes had lifts, two having more than one. Most lifts could accommodate wheelchairs but only 21 per cent could cope with a stretcher, a factor particularly worrying to staff. It is of major concern that the 1970s purpose-built homes are characterized by obstacles to mobility which are traditionally associated with older homes. Although problems associated with access to bedrooms, bathrooms, and toilets show a marked diminution in new homes, crucial areas of mobility such as manoeuvrability through doorways and along corridors continue to create difficulties for physically frail residents.

Safety

The safety of residents in care is of paramount concern to the staff and to the local authority. This is demonstrated in the staff preoccupation with watching over residents. In terms of the physical environment, safety precautions manifest themselves most dramatically in relation to fire, and in all of the hundred homes an approved fire alarm system was provided, in accordance with the 1973 Building Note and the Fire Regulations (Home Office 1983). Four out of five homes were fitted with smoke and heat detectors and in all homes firedoors were fitted along corridors, which were mainly open during the day and closed at night. Yet, in spite of these precautions, senior staff in only fifty-five homes felt that their system was adequate. Problems arose due to a lack of emergency lighting (with some staff having to resort to using torches), too few staff on duty at night, a shortage of smoke or heat detectors, and the likelihood of problems in evacuating residents from first and second floors.

Apart from fire precautions, resident safety is seen to depend on staff surveillance. However, as a mediator between resident and staff, personal alarm systems are widely used. In three-quarters of the homes, call systems were installed in both bathrooms and WCs, and in all but one home there were call systems in residents' bedrooms (*Table 9*).

Table 9 *Types of alarm systems*

	% of homes
Call system in bathroom and WC	75
Call system in bathroom only	18
Call system in WC only	2
Call system in bedrooms	99
Call system can be reached from all residents' beds in 81% of homes.	

The location of call systems in private areas of the home rather than in public areas suggests the patterns of surveillance common in the residential setting. Emphasis is placed on the congregation of residents in public areas during the day, which enables staff to keep a watching eye over residents, and at night on the provision of alternative call systems to cover for staff when few are on duty. Yet, even given the wide coverage of bedroom alarms, only 53 per cent of staff felt that the home had adequate emergency facilities in resident bedrooms. The main problems concerned resident access to the alarms in their bedrooms, the need for more flexible controls, and an easier system for locating calls once the alarm had been raised.

Daytime surveillance by staff is often facilitated by the existence of glass panels in doors and by the location of the main office within sight of the main entrance. During the night the use of lights enables staff to observe resident behaviour. With the exception of three homes, all bedroom corridors were lit at night, and in a third all or some resident bedrooms were lit by night-lights, with lights over the wash-basin sometimes used where night-lights were not provided.

Very few homes enable residents to lock their bedroom doors. In all cases this practice was justified by staff as a safety precaution. In some homes locks were provided, but it was often reported that keys had been lost and that residents could not be trusted with keys. In contrast to bedrooms, most bathrooms and WCs could be locked from the inside and there were emergency unlocking arrangements to enable staff to assist a resident who needed help. It is interesting that this principle was not applied to bedrooms.

The importance placed on safety in residential homes relates to anxiety about risk-taking. This in itself stems from the responsibility vested in local authorities whereby they are accountable for the lives of individuals. For example, a dilemma arises with regard to the policy and practice concerning residents bringing to the home large items of furniture. In three-quarters of the homes, all or some resident bedrooms had fixed furniture, especially fitted wardrobes. This arrangement was explained as an attempt to eliminate the danger of residents' pulling a heavy item of furniture down on top of themselves, or that some old people's furniture from home would be worm-infested and unsuitable, and finally that the local authority did not have anywhere to store excess furniture. These explanations serve to support practices which minimize risk-taking and expressions of individuality, and emphasize safety and block treatment.

Community integration

The integration of the residential home within the local community depends not only on the involvement of local people within the home but also on the participation of residents and staff outside the home. Staff are predominantly local people who live near to the home and are part of the local community, but what about the residents? Of the thousand residents interviewed, half did not go out of the home at all, although the more mobile male residents were far more active than the women. Those residents who went out were asked about trips to places like the post office, local shops, the doctor, the cinema, church, the pub, and bingo. Those who did not go out were asked whether they would like the opportunity to visit such places. The most popular destination was the local shops, followed by the pub and the post office for men, and the post office and the church for women. The greatest need from those who were 'homebound' came from women who wanted to go to the local shops and to church, reflecting residents' desire to undertake 'normal' activities.

While age, sex, health, and mobility are all key factors determining community participation, the proximity of local amenities and ease of access are also important. The 1973 Building Note offers the following guidance on the siting of homes:

> 'Sites should be reasonably level, access to roads and public transport and to ordinary amenities of town or village life – shops, post office, churches and places of entertainment – should be easy and distances short.'   (DHSS and Welsh Office 1973: 2)

In most cases efforts had been made to site homes within relatively easy access of facilities and many were sited within a quarter to half a mile of amenities. However, there is evidence to show that even this distance may be too great and that, unless facilities were within a few hundred yards of the home, residents had extreme difficulty getting there unassisted. The only exceptions were visits to clubs, church, or relatives, where residents were usually collected by car:

> 'Most of the visitors come in their own cars. My grandson comes by car, he came all day yesterday. We had our lunch in town, and

then he took me down by the river all afternoon. That was lovely, that was. I can get in the car, we have to lift my legs sometimes because I'm a bit awkward, but I get in.'

or the occasional resident who hired a taxi to go to the shops or on a special visit:

'We had another hairdresser here and she had to finish because she was having a baby. So I had a taxi and went down to Anderton Street, and then came back up.'

The location studies also gave some support to the view that residents who lived in the neighbourhood of the home prior to admission were most likely to maintain activities outside the home. However, while familiarity and accessibility may be important factors in terms of participation, they cannot compensate for a lack of mobility, and it is only the most mobile residents who manage to interact with the local community independently. Residents cannot rely on staff to help them to maintain their links with the community.

Staff views of residents' activities outside the home at the same time condemn and defend; the consensus was that the majority of residents did not move out of the building though there were residents whom they felt could 'go out, but didn't'. They commented: 'It's not that they can't [go out]; they won't', and, 'Some of them can't move, but the majority, they just don't want to.' However, in some respects, resident apathy is reinforced by the protective attitudes of staff to residents' disabilities and the need to minimize risk-taking. Observations showed that on occasion residents who were fairly active outside the home were told 'not to overdo it' and were advised not to go out too often as this could affect their health.

This dual role of staff as protector and facilitator is seen in relation to many aspects of resident activity. In most homes staff stated that there were no rules and regulations governing residents going out of the building, and yet the location studies showed that all residents informed staff before going out. This was said to be both for the residents' safety and so that staff could organize mealtimes more efficiently. Staff commented:

'We need to know when and where residents are going but there are no restrictions on coming or going.'

Given that half the residents interviewed said that they did not go outside the grounds of the home, other ways are explored to try and involve residents in the world outside. In many homes the staff organize activities to take residents out of the home, and the annual or twice-yearly outings to the seaside or country park have been common practice in most homes. In many homes these one-day outings are being replaced by shorter, local visits for smaller groups, when residents can revisit local pubs and beauty spots or attend a show. Nevertheless, as with so many activities in residential homes, these trips are commonly organized for residents by staff. While a residents' committee may be involved in some homes, in others there is little joint decision-making.

For many residents, the reality of the 'community' is reduced to a view from the window or activities seen from the grounds of the home. Many residents said that they sat in the grounds of the home, weather permitting. Staff often persuade residents to go outside on a fine day, but in some cases they face stiff opposition as residents complain of being too cold, or that it is too windy. Often this is due to the poor design of sitting areas and a failure to see the grounds of the home as a potential recreational area for residents.

Given the vagaries of the British weather, for many residents the outside world becomes that which they can only sit and watch from the inside. Yet there is evidence that the layout of some residential lounges may deny residents the opportunity to 'watch the world go by'. The positioning of lounge seating and the height of window sills have important implications for visual contact with the outside world. Given that links with the wider community may facilitate the adjustment to institutional settings (Rowles 1981), this lack of stimulation may be important.

At the beginning of this chapter we asked whether the residential home had been built for the residents or staff. As with so many public buildings, it appears that the architects have worked from design guidance. They do not often consult the users to learn at 'first hand' what old people need. Successive Building Notes have used the analogy of domestic housing while at the same time setting institutional standards. Our description of spatial arrangements begins to confirm the reality of the home as an institution where the needs of the organization have to be met. In this case the physical environment has not been designed to take account of residents' lifestyles, other than at a prosthetic level. In contrast, design functions only at the level at which staff control and physically care for residents, as highlighted in the discussion of the realities of privacy, autonomy, negotiability, safety, and community integration. This function of residential care is also demonstrated historically. In recent years there has been a recognition of the need to increase provision of private bedroom space, and yet the provision of public space has been maintained. We would argue that this failure, in terms of design, to shift the balance of residential life whole-heartedly in favour of the individual is further evidence of the strength of institutional forces and the illusion of domesticity.

Note

1. While 62 per cent of the thousand respondents in the survey had a single room, only 50 per cent of all residents in the hundred homes had a single room. This discrepancy arises from the necessity to substitute some of the residents originally sampled and one characteristic of this process appears to be the greater likelihood of the substitutes having a single rather than a shared room. The original sample were more likely to be mentally or physically frail and it appears that these residents also more commonly shared rooms than had a room to themselves.

CHAPTER 6

Institutional living

At this point in the analysis we have assembled all the components of residential care. We have noted how the design of homes has been undertaken against a background of competing ideologies, the historical weight of the institution versus the rhetoric of domesticity and family care. In the midst of this conflict we find the residential staff caught between the professional role of paramedic or social worker and the kinship role of extended family. At the same time elderly residents, predominantly old women, are relocated from familiar surroundings to a 'home' from home. Given these fundamental contradictions we ask what are the effects of institutional living and whether or not variation exists between homes. Are some homes less institutional than others? And if so, does this affect the well-being of residents? Particular attention is paid to a recent innovation in residential care, small group living, where the ideals of interdependency, resident autonomy, and self-help are highlighted. It is amongst these homes that we might expect to find the most progressive practice. We also consider how the realities of residential life compare to an 'ideal' setting as perceived by residents, thus enabling us to look forward to the care settings of the future. First, however, we must consider what is already known about institutionalization, how this has been studied, and which findings relate particularly to the care of old people.

Theoretical perspectives on institutional settings

A number of important empirical studies of the residential life of old people in local authority homes have been undertaken in Britain in recent years (Booth 1985; Booth *et al*. 1983a, 1983b; Evans *et al*. 1981; Wade, Sawyer, and Bell 1983; Godlove, Richard, and Rodwell 1982). However, relatively few attempts have been made to develop a model of the residential process and its outcome for the lives of elderly people (see Davies and Knapp 1981; Booth 1985). A review of the literature shows that most theoretical work in this area has come from the USA where a number of complementary themes emerge from the disciplines of psychology and sociology, converging in what can be described as interactionist, transactional, and ecological perspectives. Three specific areas of research can be identified – first that which builds on the work of Goffman (1961) and his essays on 'total institutions'; second, the work of Kleemeier (1959, 1961) and the development of models of 'congruence' between person and environment (Kahana, 1974); and third, the related tradition of social ecology associated with Lawton (1970) and Moos (1974, 1980).

In *Asylums* Goffman (1981) focuses on the similarities between institutions rather than their differences, and presents an abstracted ideal of 'institutional totality' against which reality can be measured. In doing so he identifies four main characteristics that distinguish 'total institutions', which he defines as follows:

'First, all aspects of life are conducted in the same place and under the same single authority. Second, each phase of the member's daily activity is carried on in the immediate company of a large batch of others, all of whom are treated alike and required to do the same things together. Third, all phases of the day's activities are tightly scheduled, with one activity leading at a pre-arranged time into the next, the whole sequence of activities being imposed from above by a system of explicit formal rulings and a body of officials. Finally, the various enforced activities are brought together into a single rational plan purportedly designed to fulfil the official aims of the institution.'   (Goffman 1961: 17)

Subsequently, researchers have sought to identify the degree to which these aspects of institutional regime are found within their own particular field of study (for example mental hospitals, Wing and Brown 1970; hostels, Apte 1968), and in 1968 King and Raynes developed the Resident Management Practices Scale for use in children's homes (King, Raynes, and Tizard, 1971). This schedule, after Goffman, distinguished four dimensions of institutional life which varied between settings: the rigidity of the routine, the block treatment of inmates, the depersonalization of inmates, and the social distance between staff and inmates, which Goffman had termed 'binary management'. In order to highlight the extent to which the staff and the resident worlds could become separate, they also defined settings as 'institution oriented' or 'child oriented'. Institution oriented settings were characterized by greater social distance between residents and staff. This was developed further by Raynes, Pratt, and Roses (1979) in a study of institutions for the mentally handicapped. Thus settings were defined as resident oriented or institutionally oriented, as one of four dimensions of care. Other measures were used to identify the characteristics of the physical environment, the degree of community contact and aspects of staff speech as an indication of the type of communication between staff and residents.

In relation to institutional settings for old people, the work of Bennett and colleagues in developing an 'index of totality', provided an early application of Goffman's work (Bennett and Nahemow 1965) and in Britain, Townsend and Kimbell (1975), using a modified version of the King and Raynes Scale, studied the regime characteristics of ten residential homes in the former county of Cheshire, focusing on the 'structure of routine', 'depersonalization', and 'social distance' and their relationship with residents' characteristics. Their findings revealed no relationship between measures of resident dependency and regime characteristics, although there was a positive association between levels of mental confusion and the number of activities engaged in, and a negative association between levels of mental confusion and social distance (Townsend and Kimbell, 1975: 2,286). However, the researchers comment that they cannot make 'statements of cause and effect', the direction of causality being unproven.

At the same time as Goffman was concerned with 'institutional totality', Robert Kleemeier had already begun to define the characteristics of special settings for older people in terms of psychological constructs. In presenting a transactional view of person and residential environment he identified three main continuums within the institutional milieu:

Segregation/non-segregation The extent to which members are differentiated from non-members (i.e. degree to which residents are homogeneous in terms of age-group, sex, health status, level of functioning).

Institutional control/non-institutional control The extent to which administration and staff determine resident behaviour, rather than resident self-determination; the degree to which the resident must adapt her lifestyle in order to meet these forms of social control.

Congregation/non-congregation The extent to which members do everything at the same time. The degree of privacy is an essential component of congregation. (Kleemeier 1961: 273)

Such concepts are similar to Goffman's 'batch living' and 'binary management' (1961) and other authors, notably Pincus (1968a, 1968b) and Kahana (1974), have developed these themes both at the level of conceptualization and evaluation. Pincus developed the Home for the Aged Description Questionnaire (HDQ) focusing on twelve dimensions of residential life. Three main aspects of the institutional setting were identified: the physical plant; rules, regulations, and programme; and staff behaviour with residents; and each of these areas was considered in relation to the dimensions: public/private, structured/unstructured, resource sparse/resource rich, and isolated/integrated (Pincus 1968b). Although the HDQ was originally designed to be completed by staff, in a later study interviews were carried out with both residents and staff and responses compared (Pincus and Wood 1970). Their findings showed that not only did staff and resident perceptions of the institutional environment vary but also that different residents expect and desire different things from the environment (Pincus and Wood 1970). Such conflicting viewpoints are obviously of importance if we are to understand the totality of residential life and the various perspectives of residents and staff in our own data are discussed later in this chapter.

Like Pincus, Kahana has also built upon Kleemeier's original concepts in her congruence model of person–environment interaction. Here both individual needs and environmental characteristics are measured in relation to seven dimensions: segregation, congregation, control, and four dimensions based on characteristics of the aged individual, stimulation/engagement, structure, effect, and impulse control. Multivariate analysis is used to determine whether outcome measured in terms of satisfaction and morale can be predicted by the discrepancy or congruence between individual needs and the environment. Such findings enable the researcher to suggest how adjustment could be made to accommodate any discrepancies. In a study of three homes for the aged, Kahana was able to show that congruence between individuals' needs and the environment emerged as important and significant determinants of morale (Kahana 1974: 200).

Kahana acknowledges that her model of congruence has its origins in earlier ecological traditions where human behaviour is seen as a function of the relationship between person and environment (Kahana 1974: 183; Lewin 1935; Murray 1938). Such work also forms the basis of the social ecology model of ageing developed by Lawton and colleagues at the Philadelphia Geriatric Centre (Lawton and Nahemow 1973) and the work of Moos and colleagues at the Social Ecology Laboratory, Palo Alto, California (Moos *et al.* 1979; Lemke *et al.* 1979). In developing their model of environmental press, Lawton and colleagues also argue that a relationship exists between the competence of the individual in terms of biological health, cognitive skill, and ego strength, and the demands or press of the settings in which the person behaves (Lawton 1980). Hence some environments are said to make more demands on the individual than others and, whereas some residents may cope and adjust, others will not.

Consequent upon this model is the 'environmental docility hypothesis' that 'the less competent the individual, the greater the impact of environmental factors on that individual' (Lawton 1980: 14). While one may crudely equate this concept with the fact that older people with increasingly frail health require a more supportive environment, as the author points out, the meaning of competence is far more complex. Lawton's model also allows for certain tolerance levels with regard to press. He argues that on the one hand a certain level of press creates a tension through which the individual may experience growth.

On the other hand, the residential environment may exert too few demands on the elderly person, leading to maladaptive behaviour such as boredom and apathy.

We would suggest that the range of adaptive behaviour demonstrated by elderly residents will not be uniform and that the impact of the institutional environment is multi-faceted, being functional, personal (emotional), and symbolic. For instance, a residential home without a lift may create problems for an old person with mobility problems; a shared bedroom may be appreciated by some residents as long as the sharer does not make the arrangement intolerable; the very fact of living within an environment known as an old people's home may affect well-being.

Finally Moos and colleagues (1979), also working within the ecological tradition, have developed a series of schedules for evaluating care settings for old people. Their approach has been to identify the unique nature of different environments along a number of dimensions and once again to establish the degree of fit between individual and setting. This has culminated in the development of the Multi-phasic Environmental Assessment Procedure (MEAP) which is based on four conceptual domains: resident and staff resources, policy and programme resources, social climate resources, and physical and architectural resources (Lemke *et al.* 1979). Of particular interest to this study are the Physical and Architectural Features Checklist (PAF) and the Sheltered Care Environment Scale. A multi-method approach to data collection is adopted in the MEAP in a similar way to that undertaken in the National Consumer Study. Thus aspects of the physical environment are recorded by direct observation and the PAF assesses nine dimensions of physical and architectural resources, focusing on the availability of such resources rather than their utilization.

In contrast, the Sheltered Care Environment Scale aims to collect information from residents and staff concerning seven dimensions of institutional life: cohesion and conflict (as indicators of the relationships between residents and staff), independence and self-exploration (which relate to whether or not residents experience room for personal growth and self-determination), and organization, resident influence, and physical comfort (which provide indicators of the overall social or organizational climate of the institution). Residents and staff are asked to complete both a 'Real Form' – relating to how they perceive the present social environment within the facility – and an 'Ideal Form', which asks them to envisage their ideal sheltered care facility. A comparison can therefore be made between resident and staff views and between real and ideal perceptions. The degree of congruence or discontinuity between real and ideal perceptions enables the researcher to comment on the degree of person–environment fit for individuals and groups of residents. Their analysis has shown the complexity of the social environment of sheltered care settings, with the type of facility, physical and architectural policy and programme characteristics, and resident and staff characteristics all being influential (Moos and Igra 1980; Lemke and Moos 1980). They have also demonstrated that cohesion, independence, and self-exploration are positively related to the size of the facility, while little relationship is seen with staff–resident ratios.

The work of psychologists such as Lawton, Moos, and Kahana allows us a greater insight into individual response and adaptation to institutionalization, as well as into the collective response of residents as a group. Such research also provides a basis for developing a broader framework for understanding the residential process. Davies and Knapp (1981), in utilizing a production function approach to the study of old people's homes, offer one such framework. They focus on the inputs and outputs of care and the relationships between them. Inputs are classified under three headings: resource inputs, including fixed capital and manpower; non-resource inputs, the various aspects of the social environment; and quasi-inputs, pertaining to individual characteristics of residents. They view output mainly in terms of the general well-being of residents (psychological well-being, morale, life satisfaction, engagement) although outcomes such as mortality, morbidity, and the impact of residential care for residents' significant-others are also examined. Such a model is in many ways similar to the one being developed here, and in the following section we examine just how residential homes differ and what this means for elderly residents.

A variety of settings

In order to assess whether or not variation exists between the hundred homes in the study it was necessary to develop a series of summary indicators for aspects of the social and physical environments. A review of the literature shows that certain dimensions of the social environment have been identified as of particular importance. First, the degree to which residents can live a more or less individual lifestyle as indicated by the availability of privacy and choice within the home, and the scope for resident autonomy and self-determination. Second, the locus of control, within the home; whether this is geared towards the needs of residents or staff. Such factors are demonstrated by the organizational practices of the home and are structured by rules and regulations. They are also related to the less tangible area of staff attitudes and personality of the officer in charge and his or her particular style of operating (Sinclair 1971). However, such factors are difficult to measure and to some extent fall outside the scope of this study. Instead, we have focused on that aspect of the social environment relating to organizational practices and staff responses to questions concerning resident self-determination and participation within the home to enable us to derive indicators of institutional regime. Twenty-eight items completed by senior staff on both the local authority postal questionnaire and the staff questionnaire were used to develop four additive scales as indicators of various characteristics of regime (see Appendix 2). They are defined as follows:

Choice/freedom   Degree to which residents have a choice or degree of freedom over their lifestyle, e.g. mealtimes, going out, getting up.

Privacy   Availability of privacy – both personal and in interactions with others.

Involvement   Degree of resident participation in the organization of home life. Their knowledge concerning how the home is run.

Engagement/stimulation   Degree to which staff encourage resident autonomy and independence.

High scores on all these items indicate a more progressive style of organization within the home, with the emphasis on residents being treated as individuals with some control over their lives.

In the earlier discussion of the physical environment we focused on the impact of particular aspects of design for the lives of residents. Yet such themes may also be developed as summary indicators which give some indication of both form and function. As a detailed inspection was carried out on each of the hundred homes in the sample, data was available to assess the physical environment along eight of the nine dimensions defined by Moos and colleagues in their Physical and Architectural Checklist (1979). Guided by this work, eight additive scales were developed which tap key dimensions of the physical environment within the context of British old people's homes (see Appendix 2). They are defined as follows:

Physical amenities   are those features of the environment which add convenience or increase comfort, e.g. if there is a WC for both male and female residents within the recommended 10 metres of both dining-room and lounges; if bedside lights are provided.

Social–recreational aids   give an indication of facilities which encourage recreational activities or increased social interaction, e.g. where there is more than one television; if chairs are provided in the main entrance hall.

Prosthetic aids and orientational aids   assess degree to which physical environment enables residents to negotiate the setting and to carry out some activities of daily living without necessarily being dependent on staff, e.g. prosthetic aids – WCs adapted for wheelchair users; orientational aids – presence of a notice board.

Safety features   are not only a form of security for residents but also for staff, e.g. call system in bedrooms, bathrooms, and WCs.

Architectural choice   includes items relating to environmental control and choice, e.g. whether residents can open the windows in lounges or control heating in their bedrooms; whether residents have somewhere to lock away personal possessions in their own rooms.

Space availability   assesses the average amount of public and private space available for residents using the design guidance given in the 1973 Building Note.

Staff facilities   consider the present facilities for staff, e.g. if staff have their own WC; whether or not a duty room is provided.

(See Moos and Lemke 1980)

An assessment was not undertaken concerning Moos' ninth dimension: 'community accessibility' as insufficient data were collected at the site of each of the hundred homes.

In addition to these dimensions, two further summary scales – resident oriented, staff oriented – were derived which incorporate aspects of both the physical and social environments and describe a home in terms of whether or not the residential setting facilitates staff or resident actions. The main parameters of these fourteen dimensions are given in *Table 10*. In order to compare these different dimensions both within and between homes, average scores for each dimension were converted to a base of 100. As the table shows, there is considerable variability between the different dimensions.

Table 10   *Dimensions of the social and physical environments*

	maximum score	range	$\bar{x}$	sd	$\bar{x}$ score
choice	11	2–10	6.7	1.9	61
privacy	5	0–4	2.3	0.9	47
involvement	6	0–6	1.7	1.5	28
engagement/stimulation	7	1–6	3.2	1.1	45
physical amenities	19	8–19	13.6	2.1	72
social–recreational amenities	8	2–8	5.1	1.1	64
prosthetic aids	14	2–11	8.3	1.7	59
orientation aids	5	0–5	1.8	1.0	36
safety features	14	4–14	10.8	1.8	77
architectural choice	20	4–18	13.1	2.8	55
space availability	3	0–3	1.6	1.0	53
staff facilities	7	3–7	5.7	3.2	81
resident oriented	17	2–17	9.6	2.8	56
staff oriented	12	0–12	6.2	2.3	52

Scores base = 100

In terms of physical environment highest mean scores were seen for staff facilities and safety features, aspects of design which can be said to reflect the institutional nature of residential homes. General physical amenities also achieved high scores, with slightly lower scores for those aspects of the physical environment which may be considered as enhancing the lifestyle of residents, that is social–recreational amenities, prosthetic aids, architectural choice, and space availability. In relation to regime characteristics, the dimension concerning choice has the highest score while, in contrast, resident involvement in the affairs of the homes achieves a very low score.

In order to look at between-homes differences, analysis was undertaken in relation to five main variables: age of home (date at which the home opened as a residential home for the elderly), building type (whether purpose built, conversion, or conversion with modern extension), number of beds, organization (in terms of group, semi-group, or non-group living), and home-type (using the typology outlined in Chapter 5 where homes are defined in terms of both internal complexity of layout and size, that is small and simple, medium and semi-complex, large and complex). (See *Table 11*.)

As expected, some advances in the provision of physical resources are reflected in the age, building type, and size of home. Purpose built homes, those with between forty and sixty residents and those opened in the 1960s and to some extent the 1970s, were more likely to score well on physical amenities, social–recreational, and prosthetic aids and offer greater architectural choice. Those homes classed as small and simple in terms of organization and design fared badly in relation to most dimensions of physical environment, with the exception of physical amenities and space availability. This is not surprising given that a number of old adapted properties fell into this category.

Variation was also seen in relation to organizational style. Although non-group homes displayed fairly average profiles, differences were apparent between the small sub-samples of group (N = 11) and semi-group homes (N = 12). For all dimensions of the physical environment, semi-group homes revealed average or above average scores, and as such can be said to be the most resource-rich environments. Particularly high scores were obtained for prosthetic and orientational aids, safety features, and space availability. The semi-group homes in this sample, though predominantly purpose built, were not designed for group living. The reorganization of space by staff often resulted in partial grouping with either the formation of one or two groups which sat and ate their meals separately from the other residents or with grouped lounges but a communal dining-room. Thus residents benefited from greater space availability. Orientational aids were more prevalent in these homes, especially the use of signs and colour codings, both in terms of paintwork and carpeting. It may be said that the movement of residents between groups and communal areas has necessitated such directional aids; indeed the enthusiasm with which staff had adopted this new system often resulted in improvements to the physical environment, and incidentally to the social environment.

Of the eleven group homes in the study, only three had been purpose built to a group-unit design; the remainder had also been reorganized which often entailed the division of large lounges and dining-rooms into smaller group sitting/dining-rooms. In contrast to the semi-group homes, this often resulted in a total loss of communal space. These homes attained below average scores for social–recreational, prosthetic, and orientational aids, as well as for staff facilities. While purpose-built homes may boast a number of facilities such as visitors' rooms, quiet rooms, and common rooms, the reorganization of even these homes often resulted in a shortage of extra space, and staff often complained of a lack of common recreational space in group-living homes. However, in spite of these deficiencies in physical resources, the group homes did score highly in terms of architectural choice, revealing something of the relationship between organization and design.

In summary, over time, homes have become larger in both actual size and number of residents, and more complex in design, and it is these more complex buildings that are likely to offer a wider range of amenities for both residents and staff (see *Figure 7*). Homes where an attempt has been made to change the organizational structure, as in the group and semi-group living settings, also offer the potential for interaction within the built environment. Semi-group homes appear more likely to provide prosthetic environments which are both secure and negotiable, as well as rich in resources that assist staff work routines while, in contrast, group homes would seem to offer residents greater opportunity in physical terms for achieving an individual lifestyle

Table 11 Dimensions of the physical and social environment broken down by characteristics of home type

Dimension	non-group home	semi-group home	group home	small and simple	medium and semi-complex	large and complex	purpose-built	conversion	conversion and extension	pre-1959	1960-69	post-1970	< 30 residents	30-39 residents	40-49 residents	50 or more residents	$\bar{x}$
physical amenities	72	73	73	74	71	72	73	69	70	70	73	71	76	69	73	70	72
social-recreational aids	64	63	59	59	65	64	64	64	58	60	65	63	55	66	65	57	64
prosthetic aids	58	66	56	50	59	63	63	43	48	47	61	63	47	56	62	59	59
orientational aids	36	48	33	30	36	41	39	28	33	28	35	45	23	38	36	43	36

Table 11 *contd.*

safety features	77	81	79	73	76	81	80	66	75	69	80	78	59	75	79	83	77
architectural choice	64	67	72	57	64	72	69	58	58	52	66	73	52	62	67	70	66
space availability	50	67	54	58	52	50	52	44	63	50	53	54	62	67	48	44	53
staff facilities	76	80	77	72	77	79	78	70	72	70	75	83	63	77	78	78	81
choice	58	65	73	61	59	58	59	59	65	64	58	63	57	60	63	56	61
privacy	45	48	58	49	40	40	40	43	56	48	46	47	42	44	52	42	47
involvement	26	25	39	29	19	32	27	31	24	31	28	26	38	28	30	18	28
engagement/ stimulation	44	54	48	46	44	45	47	45	46	46	42	50	54	43	44	49	45
resident-oriented environment	55	64	61	56	55	58	54	57	58	56	56	57	51	58	57	55	56
staff-oriented environment	52	56	43	51	49	53	54	50	52	54	52	50	53	53	50	55	52
N =	77	12	11	75	12	12	18	48	33	16	49	35	7	25	48	20	

Scores base = 100

Figure 7 Variation in dimensions of the physical environment within four
residential homes

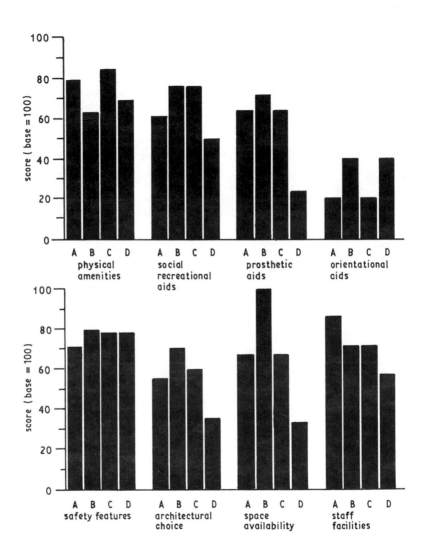

A – purpose built, traditional   C – purpose built, semi-group living
B – purpose built, group living   D – adapted with modern extension,
                                            traditional

through a higher level of environmental control.

Consideration of organizational practice, however, complicates this picture. An examination of mean scores gives some indication that the more recently built, large and complex homes in the sample were characterized by staff who encouraged choice and privacy for residents, which may reflect exposure to new ideas in caring practices. However, small and simple homes also scored highly in terms of choice, privacy, and resident involvement, although it is also the case that these older and smaller homes were more likely to offer a staff oriented environment than one geared predominantly to resident self-determination. Homes operating the group-living system had high scores for all dimensions with the exception of staff orientation, where scores were particularly low. In contrast, semi-group homes scored especially well in terms of resident engagement and stimulation, while at the same time appearing to offer an environment that, to some extent, offered a compromise between meeting resident and staff needs.

Thus, although the physical design of homes may reveal certain patterns over time, trends in the development of more liberal organizational practices are far less tangible. Variation in the characteristics of the social environment for any one home is demonstrated by *Figure 8*, which again considers the four homes identified in *Figure 7*, each home having certain strengths and weaknesses. By focusing on individual homes, our analysis confirms the work of Booth who states that the differences *between* homes in the way they are run are more than matched by variations *within* homes (Booth 1985: 168). The identification of what he terms 'multiple regimes' is important, for it highlights the complexity of operational policy, with few homes capable of being labelled extremely liberal or extremely authoritarian. The reasons for variation in the characteristics of operational style within homes are numerous, including, no doubt, the philosophy of care, the attitudes and awareness of staff to residents' needs, the design of the building, the relationship between senior and care staff, staff shift work, and the characteristics of the resident group.

Correlations between the dimensions of the social environment and other indicators of home life reveal not only the associations between the social and the physical environments, but also the characteristics of resident and staff groups. It is not surprising that both privacy and choice

Figure 8   Variation in dimensions of organizational style within four
residential homes

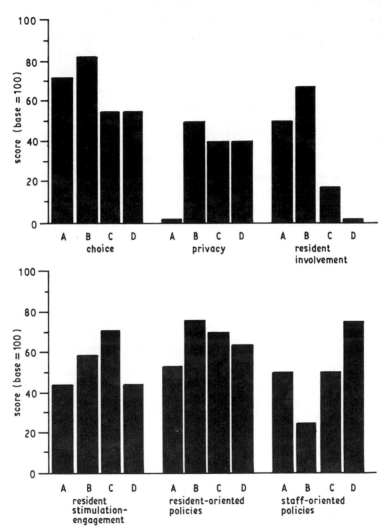

A – purpose built, traditional   C – purpose built, semi-group living
B – purpose built, group living   D – adapted with modern extension,
                                          traditional

should be associated with homes that provide a resource-rich environment for residents with an emphasis on single bedrooms and amenities that facilitate resident autonomy. Of perhaps greater interest is that resident oriented environments and those that offer greater opportunity for stimulation/engagement show a negative association with the proportion of mentally infirm residents in the home ($r = -0.29$, $p < 0.01$; $r = -0.20$, $p < 0.02$ respectively) whereas the level of physical impairment amongst residents is associated positively with staff oriented environments ($r = 0.21$, $p < 0.01$). While we cannot state with certainty the cause and effect of such relationships, various explanations are possible. Thus group homes, which we have noted as resident-oriented environments, also had a lower percentage of mentally infirm residents than other homes in the sample, which may be due to particular admission policies. Such findings confirm those of Evans *et al.* (1981) who found that more institutionally oriented practices were associated with higher levels of mental and physical impairment amongst residents.

There is also some evidence that the characteristics of the staff group affect resident behaviour. However, the nature of this relationship is far from clear-cut. Whereas a negative association exists between the number of staff and levels of resident participation in the wider organization of the home ($r = -0.20$, $p < 0.02$), there is a positive association between staff encouragement of resident autonomy and staff/resident ratios ($r = 0.20$, $p < 0.02$).

Our analysis has established that variation does exist both within and between the hundred homes with regard to both the physical environment and operational policy. Yet, although the former is indisputable, the latter is less clear-cut. While we can distinguish variation on the basis of staff accounts, we are still left with an overall impression, supported by our observations, that residential life, whatever the setting, is predominantly public and communal, routinized and impersonal. These conflicting accounts may reflect a mismatch between stated policy and actual practice, but if so, why is this the case? We may come closer to answering this question if we can establish whether residents and staff living and working in different types of settings are more or less content, in other words whether the variation in setting and operational style affects outcome.

How content are residents and staff?

Can we assess whether the type of residential setting has any effect on the well-being of residents and staff or are such factors insignificant when compared to the impact of past circumstances, health, and life outside the home? Certainly the work of authors such as Tobin and Lieberman (1976) provides important evidence for believing that major changes in well-being for elderly people occur prior to admission, once the decision has been made to seek institutional care. If this is true, then variation in the type of residential setting may have little impact on the lives of elderly residents or it may prove impossible to disentangle the factors at work before and after admission.

In order to assess the impact of different types of residential homes on the lives of residents and staff, we need to try to establish some way of measuring outcome. To date, two forms of measurement have commonly been used by researchers: first, subjective indicators of psychological well-being, morale, happiness, or perceived satisfaction with life, and second, more objective indicators such as levels of personal functioning and rates of morbidity and mortality (Davies and Knapp 1981). In terms of resident outcome, the latter are obviously fairly stable measures in terms of data collection as they do not involve the researcher in trying to elicit or interpret the complexities of subjective feelings (see Booth 1985). Yet as indicators of quality of life in institutional settings they may prove too simplistic and less sensitive in identifying the subtleties of residential life. Such measures may also be largely predetermined by other factors, notably health and past circumstances. Do high rates of mortality or morbidity reflect the quality of care in a particular home or are they totally dependent on the health of residents prior to admission? Are high activity levels amongst residents indicative of enhanced well-being or do they merely reflect the operational policy of a particular type of regime? In a recent publication Booth has been forced to conclude that the residential environment has very little influence on outcome measured in terms of both mortality and morbidity (Booth 1985: 179).

In the case of more subjective measures, the most common forms of measurement used in studies of older people, such as the Philadelphia Geriatric Morale Scale (Lawton 1972, 1975), the Life Satisfaction Index

(Neugarten, Havighurst, and Tobin 1961) and the Affect Balance Scale (Bradburn and Caplovitz 1965; Bradburn 1969) have been developed in the USA on non-institutional samples. By using such measures, or even more general questions concerning satisfaction with older people in institutional settings, we are beset not only with difficulties in explanation (Peace, Hall, and Hamblin 1979) but also in interpretation of findings and their validity. There is a tendency for residents to express high levels of satisfaction with their new environment (see Chapter 3) which may reflect a willingness to comply with the norms of the institution from a position of dependency (Bland and Bland 1983; Booth 1983). Even where variation in response does occur it is impossible to disentangle whether such positive or negative feelings are due to present circumstances, to what happened to the older person prior to admission to care, to current state of health, or to some aspects of the individual's personality. We would therefore agree with Booth that measures of well-being, morale, and perceived satisfaction do not enable us to distinguish between the experience of care and the outcome of care (1985: 103) for elderly patients and we hope that such findings will be treated with caution. With respect to staff, the use of such indicators are perhaps less problematic, although staff job satisfaction and psychological well-being are possibly intimately related and, as we have seen, neither is determined solely by the environment in which staff work.

Nevertheless, while recognizing these limitations, the study set out to elicit the views of the consumer and, because of this, the feelings of residents and staff concerning their present lifestyle were deemed important. As noted in Chapter 3, a variety of questions was used to try to examine residents' feelings of well-being and satisfaction with life, both now and prior to admission, their current worries, and how they had adjusted to home life. The following variables may therefore be used as indicators of the feelings expressed by residents about home life and their current self-esteem, alongside measures of staff job satisfaction and well-being.

Table 12 Aspects of resident and staff well-being to home types

residents	non-group home	semi-group home	group home	purpose built	conversion	conversion and extension	pre-1959	1960-69	post-1970	small and simple	medium and semi-complex	large and complex	< 30 residents	30-39 residents	40-49 residents	50 or more residents	$\bar{x}$
adjustment to home	77	80	79	81	79	79	77	77	85	77	75	86	77	78	78	78	78
adjustment to ageing	56	62	54	57	63	59	59	58	57	60	57	58	60	58	57	59	58

Table 12 *contd.*

worry	16	18	24	18	16	16	16	18	20	14	18	0	16	16	18	22	18
worry about home	10	6	18	10	6	8	8	10	12	6	10	12	8	8	10	12	10
dissatisfaction since admission	47	49	50	49	40	48	47	50	45	48	49	45	48	48	48	47	48
dissatisfaction with staff/resident relations	19	19	23	20	17	18	18	19	21	14	20	21	10	16	21	24	20
staff																	
job satisfaction	75	78	70	75	75	76	75	75	76	76	75	74	74	76	75	73	75
well-being	74	74	64	72	73	74	73	73	71	71	72	73	69	73	72	74	73
worry	14	10	21	15	14	14	12	14	17	13	16	12	15	15	15	13	14
worry about home	13	6	23	14	12	12	9	12	19	9	18	10	13	10	15	15	14

Scores base = 100

The feelings of residents and staff

Residents

Adjustment to home life Resident's level of adjustment when first admitted to the home – living with others; making friends; getting to know staff; orientation. High values indicate positive adjustment.

Adjustment to ageing Adapted from Abrams Adjustment to Ageing Scale (Abrams 1978). Measure of psychological well-being. High values indicate positive well-being.

Worry Measure of resident's present anxieties or worries (adapted from Srole *et al.* 1962)

Worried about aspects of home life Factor analysis of the worry scale produced a sub-scale which taps resident's worry about aspect of home life, e.g. safety, security, home organization, and difficult relations with other residents.

Dissatisfaction since coming to home A combination of two questions concerning life satisfaction before and after admission to care. High values indicate a drop in the level of life satisfaction after admission.

Staff satisfaction Resident satisfaction with staff in terms of their social interaction with staff (seven-item scale). High scores indicate dissatisfaction.

Staff

Job satisfaction A sixteen-item scale concerning various aspects of working life – relations with other staff; job autonomy; working conditions.

Psychological well-being Affect Balance Scale (Bradburn 1969; Campbell, Converse, and Rogers 1976). Includes ten items, five items tapping negative affect and five positive affect.

Worry Measure of staff's present worries and anxieties (after Srole *et al.* 1962).

Worry about work Variable based on two items of the worry scale concerning relations with people at work and how things are going at work.

The main parameters of these ten dimensions are given in Appendix 2, and the intercorrelations between the variables show that significant associations exist between all measures concerning residents and all measures concerning staff. The direction of association is as expected, that is satisfaction measures are associated positively with each other but show negative correlations with worry items.

In order to extend the analysis undertaken in relation to the physical and social environments, we can now consider the feelings of residents and staff living within particular types of home. A comparison of mean scores shows that, whereas high scores for adjustment to home life were found for residents living in large modern homes, those in small homes, and more typically in converted properties, had higher levels of more general well-being as measured by the adjustment to ageing scale (*Table 12*). Only those living in semi-group homes scored highly on both measures. In contrast, even though levels of worry were very low for *all* residents, those living in group homes had higher than average worry scores. They also revealed greater dissatisfaction over their relationship with staff, which was also true of those living in large homes with more than fifty residents.

Data concerning staff reveal similar complexities. Staff well-being was higher in large homes and those run on semi-group or traditional (non-group) lines of organization. Job satisfaction was high in semi-group homes but low in group-living homes and, like residents, although staff do not score highly overall in terms of worries, higher than average worry scores were found for staff in group-living homes. Such analysis shows that we cannot assume for example that 'small equals happy'; the relationships are far more complex.

By correlating measures of well-being with aspects of the social and physical environments and characteristics of the resident and staff groups, we find that there is little direct relationship between well-being and physical environment. Indeed, there are few significant relationships between well-being and organizational practices, although it is important to note the associations between staff worry and resident-oriented policies ($r = 0.26$, $p < 0.01$), seen especially in group homes. Such findings may highlight the anxiety observed amongst staff when residents are temporarily out of sight or when the environment encourages activities involving an element of risk.

Other significant correlations are also of interest. As expected, there is some relationship between residents' subjective assessment of their health and both their adjustment to home life ($r = 0.20$, $p < 0.02$) and their level of worry ($r = -0.22$, $p < 0.01$). Resident dissatisfaction with staff–resident relations is associated with the number of residents ($r = 0.34$, $p < 0.01$) and staff ($r = 0.27$, $p < 0.01$) as well as the number of staff hours ($r = 0.33$, $p < 0.01$), which offers some support to the findings of Moos and colleagues which suggest that 'higher staffing levels may work to inhibit residents from doing things on their own and enhance the degree to which staff restrict and control residents' (Moos and Igra 1980: 96).

It is obvious from this analysis that institutional effects are not the only determinants of resident or staff well-being or satisfaction. Nevertheless there is some evidence to suggest that in environments where staff needs for some degree of routine, surveillance, and security in terms of resident safety are met, staff are less anxious and job satisfaction is higher. In environments where both resident and staff needs are recognized, such as in semi-group homes, both groups demonstrate higher levels of contentment. However, in homes where the environment has greater orientation towards residents rather than staff, as found in group-living homes, staff satisfaction is lower and resident views are mixed, showing signs of both satisfaction and dissatisfaction. How can we explain why progressive homes should be characterized by such levels of discontent? Perhaps it is the case that the capacity to criticize is a necessary precondition for changing residential homes. Given that the group-living system has been proposed to introduce not only a more manageable physical environment, but also a social environment which offers greater resident autonomy, it is important to look in more detail at this form of residential setting.

Small group living – a new panacea?

We have seen that, although homes which operate small group living may offer both an improved physical environment and an organizational style where staff have taken on board the needs of residents for privacy, choice, and a degree of personal autonomy, they are also homes where both residents and staff experience higher levels of worry and lower levels of personal or job satisfaction. It is possible, of course, that such findings are dependent upon the physical or mental health of residents, or the circumstances of their admission to residential care. Residents in the group-living homes studied were more physically impaired than those in other homes and were more likely to use mobility aids to get around and to say that their health was poor. However, they were less mentally frail than other residents, and residents in semi-group homes, where satisfaction was high and worry low, were not in markedly better health than in other homes. In terms of the circumstances surrounding admission, residents in the group-living homes were most likely to have entered care for 'legitimate' reasons such as their inability (or their spouse's) to manage in the community due to ill-health, accident, or other event. This was also true of residents in semi-group homes. While some variation obviously exists in terms of resident characteristics between the types of homes, such factors alone cannot explain the differences in outcome identified above.

The object of small group living in residential homes has been to break down both the physical and social environments into units where residents may achieve a greater degree of autonomy and control over their daily lives through the interdependency of the pseudo-family group. The idea is something of a compromise for it enables the local authority to maintain large and complex buildings while at the same time making the residents' world more manageable. Our findings show that not only were residents in group homes more likely to be engaged in everyday activities, such as helping with the washing up or making tea, but also they were more likely to interact with other residents, findings supported by other studies of group-living settings (Hitch and Simpson 1972; Thomas, Gough, and Spencerly 1979). However, there is also evidence that group living is more demanding on staff–resident relations; staff encouragement may be perceived by residents as staff telling them what to do. Moreover, the impact of a shortage of staff and staff changes may be amplified by the fragmentation of units. The organization of group-living homes is complex for it involves the careful structuring of a system which advocates flexibility and, because of this, the need to attach key workers to individual groups may be particularly important (see Thomas, Gough, and Spencerly 1979; Peace 1981). Unfortunately it is rare for five key workers to be on duty at any one time in order to cover all the groups and so this system rarely operates perfectly.

For staff, the operation of a group-living home should mean more flexibility over routines and daily practices. This may mean that staff do not always have a clear understanding of the more complex roles which for staff who work primarily at providing physical care, may be very confusing and unsettling. The group concept is not an easy one to put into practice. Care staff need constant support from senior staff, as they do from management, and there is a need for regular meetings to discuss both what is happening in the groups and how staff can best approach their work (see Peace 1981).

When we look at the interactions between staff and residents, we can see the dilemma in which many staff find themselves. In contrast with other types of homes, more senior staff in group homes felt that staff did too much for residents, whereas more care staff felt they did too little, which may reflect both their position within the home and past experience of caring. Fifty per cent of care staff in group homes reported problems with residents' wanting to spend time talking to them, and two-thirds of both senior and care staff in group homes expressed difficulties over a lack of resident cooperation, as did care staff in semi-group homes (*Table 13*). Care staff in group homes also reported that they had problems getting to know residents, and senior staff felt that relatives and other visitors wanted to spend too much time talking to them. All of these features can be linked to the group-living system and a heightened awareness amongst staff of the needs of residents and their relatives. Yet at the same time they are seen as problems rather than as necessary consequences of changes in policy.

Other problems that staff felt residents encountered with group living concerned interpersonal relations and increasing frailty. According to all staff, the most important problems involved 'personality clashes', 'arguments', and 'one person dominating the group'. These are common complaints in group settings and at present little is done in order to place individuals with compatible groups. The present solution to unsatisfactory social relationships is to move residents from one

Table 13   *Aspects of social interaction in group/non-group homes (staff responses)*

	group home		semi-group home		non-group home	
	senior staff	care staff	senior staff	care staff	senior staff	care staff
problems with	%	%	%	%	%	%
residents wanting to spend too much time talking with you	27	50	21	13	30	35
residents not cooperating when you ask them something	64	64	38	63	37	46
getting to know residents	9	23	8	17	10	11
relatives/other visitors wanting to spend too much time talking to you	32	9	13	8	18	10

(positive answers only)

group to another, and this requires a level of flexibility that may not be feasible. Group isolation was also a problem, with some residents barely venturing outside their groups. While isolation can be partially alleviated by building design, it also falls to the staff to encourage social interaction.

Staff also commented on the problems caused by residents who may be thought unsuitable for group living; they included the mentally infirm and the incontinent. Indeed the results of the visual game showed that residents in group homes strongly supported the notion of separating confused residents (they scored seventy-eight for this preference as compared with a score of fifty-nine for residents from semi-group homes and sixty-six for non-group homes). And finally there were difficulties for residents whose home was converted from a traditional style to that of small groups. In such cases residents experienced two forms of relocation, one from the community and another within the home.

For themselves, staff in group homes said that the system caused 'more work and more worry', and they commented on the need for more staff, favouritism among individuals and/or groups, staff adjustment to and training for group living, the difficulties caused by confused residents, and the need for alterations to buildings. All of these problems can be justified in one way or another and it is the range of these comments that enables us to suggest that the expressed feelings of residents and staff within different types of residential homes are to some extent dependent on the nature of the social and physical environment.

While the dissatisfaction and anxiety towards aspects of home life shown by residents and staff in group homes may be a function of their generally low levels of well-being, we would suggest that this is not the whole picture. We have already commented on many of the problems experienced by staff which may affect their job satisfaction. In relation to residents, their dissatisfaction and concern over aspects of home life may have both positive and negative characteristics, reflecting a level of tension in terms of the congruence between the resident and his or her environment, which revolves around the issues of risk-taking on the one hand and security on the other. Some residents may find the pressures of small group living too great, preferring the relative anonymity of a large group and the security offered by the more traditional home; others may be stimulated by the opportunities for self-determination but may find that the token nature of the group setting renders their activity meaningless. The group-living home, in aspiring to the domestic, does not live up to the expectations of either residents or staff for living or working environments.

This discussions leads us to agree with Booth's comments that, whereas some residential homes operate a 'holding' function, maintaining the elderly person at a particular level of functioning, other environments are more threatening and, while some residents cope well and find the experience personally rewarding, others do not (Booth 1985: 186). We would suggest that the compromise reached in semi-group homes, by providing a degree of resident autonomy within a more traditionally communal and controllable setting, may account for the higher levels of satisfaction reported in these homes by both residents and staff. Given the obvious importance of the balance between interdependent and dependent living, resident preferences for a particular style of residential environment may give us some indication of the degree of fit between their present setting and an ideal. It is to these issues that we now turn.

What do residents want?

During the course of the interviews with residents and staff, views were sought on what they thought would make an ideal home in terms of physical provision. As we have noted, eliciting consumer preferences from those already acculturized by familiar surroundings can prove difficult using traditional methods of interviewing, for the tendency is often to endorse present provision. However, some firm views did emerge, as shown in *Table 14*, and it is possible to demonstrate the level of congruence between resident preference and actual provision.

Table 14 *Resident and staff preferences for aspects of environment*

resident		staff	
77	per cent prefer a bedroom to themselves	75	per cent prefer a single bedroom for residents
17	per cent prefer to share a bedroom	11	per cent prefer shared bedrooms for residents
67	per cent prefer a bedsitter rather than just a bedroom	67	per cent prefer bedsitting rooms
63	per cent prefer carpet in their bedroom (only 15 per cent had fitted carpets or carpet tiles)		
66	per cent prefer small lounges		
49	per cent prefer chairs to be ungrouped	59	per cent prefer chairs to be grouped
40	per cent prefer an entrance hall where you can sit and watch		
57	per cent prefer a large dining-room	62	per cent prefer single large dining-room
80	per cent prefer small tables in dining-rooms		

In terms of bedroom allocation, three-quarters of residents have the kind of room they say they prefer. However, one in five residents did not have rooms in line with their stated preferences. Nearly all of these were residents currently sharing who would have preferred a single room. At the level of basic amenity, having a single room was seen as more important than the idea of a bedsitting room. Given the size and amenities available in current resident bedrooms, it appears that the main advantage of a single room lies in the opportunity for solitude rather than a scope for being 'at home', although residents' preference for carpeted bedrooms gives some indication of a desire for a level of comfort. Yet our data also reveal the presence of a hierarchy of need. Thus those residents who did not have a room of their own saw this as their first priority, those with their own room were more inclined to want a bedsitting room, and those who saw their room as a bedsitting room were most likely to be concerned about the environmental control of temperature and furniture arrangements.

In the more public areas of the home, a majority of residents expressed preferences for small lounges, a large dining-room, and a hallway where they could sit and watch the world go by. However, this pattern did vary for certain groups of residents. Physically frail residents were more likely to prefer a large lounge, reflecting perhaps both easier access and an opportunity to survey a wider range of activities. Although equal numbers of men and women preferred a hallway where they could sit and watch, this preference was sustained across the age span for male residents, while fewer very old women (over seventy-five years) revealed this preference, no doubt reflecting the greater use made of hallways by older men. In terms of dining-room preferences, a third of residents (N = 118 – only half of the sample answered these questions) did not have the kind of facility they said they would like; of this group 55 per cent took their meals in a large dining-room when they would have preferred a small one, with the remaining 45 per cent being 'frustrated' in the opposite direction. A preference for smaller dining-rooms was also associated with increased physical impairment amongst residents and such provision was more popular amongst staff, partly because this provided scope for segregating unsocial eaters. Indeed, the higher the incidence of mental impairment amongst the resident group, the lower the preference expressed for single large dining-rooms by both residents and staff.

In terms of seating arrangements in lounges, residents and staff preferences diverged. Residents were more likely to support the common pattern of ungrouped chairs, usually positioned around the walls of the lounge, while staff, no doubt influenced by current thinking on chair layout and social interaction, were more in favour of groups. Staff preferences appeared to be at odds with current practice and it was surprising that more had not been done to alter the situation. That staff commented on the failure of attempts to change chair layout, with residents moving grouped chairs back against the walls, indicates that the nurturing of resident–resident interactions demands more than mere chair rearrangement.

These findings indicate some of the difficulties which both residents and staff experienced in projecting themselves into an ideal situation without being influenced by their present setting. For residents this process is made doubly difficult by the fact that, as recipients of welfare, they feel they should not demand free choice. It was to overcome some of these difficulties that we developed an alternative research strategy to complement the interview data. The development of this technique, known as the visual game or the 'Ideal Home Game', is discussed in detail elsewhere (Willcocks 1984). However, the basic objective of the game is to use picture cards depicting key features of the residential setting to allow residents to make choices over aspects of the environment which they feel are important. The choices resulting from the game can then be examined in relation to survey data and the detailed observation and location studies.

Residents sorted the twenty-seven picture cards into three categories: 'important', 'don't know'/'don't mind', or 'unimportant', making their allocation on the basis of whether or not each item was an essential feature which every home should have. Residents subsequently ranked the five most important and five least important items. Scores were calculated for each card, which allowed for an overall ranking of all the items. Results for the full card set are shown in *Table 15* in rank order determined by overall consumer choice.

The top five choices were (i) safeguard against fire, (ii) windows which you can open, (iii) easily opened doors, (iv) a single bedroom, and (v) ordinary baths. The least popular items, starting from the bottom, were (i) provision of alcohol, (ii) a shared bedroom, (iii) living in groups, (iv) moveable bedroom furniture, and (v) a low-intensity night-light.

Such results appear to show that, with the exception of the 'safeguard against fire' care, residents chose aspects of the environment that were normal, unexceptional, and non-institutional; basic environmental features found in community housing. There is some indication that residents wish to maintain an element of control over their immediate physical environment, particularly in relation to temperature – that is, they want the privacy of a single room and the familiarity of an 'ordinary' bath, aspects of everyday life which were taken for granted in their former home. In contrast, aspects of

Table 15　*Ranked visual game choices: age-sex distribution (first sort)*

	men under 85 years	85 or more	women under 85 years	85 or more
safeguard against fire	93	94	92	92
windows which you can open	85	78	85	82
easily opened doors	85	79	84	82
a single room	82	80	79	83
ordinary bath	84	83	79	79
storage space	81	73	81	76
views of gardens	75	66	79	76
receiving friends in bedroom	63	63	73	78
easily identified rooms	72	63	74	66
a shop selling food/sweets/stationery	69	53	71	70
control over bedroom radiators	69	70	69	66
separate room for confused residents	65	65	67	66
different types of chair for different people	68	67	66	59
good sound insulation between rooms	64	58	64	58
a power-point in the bedroom	63	68	62	55
a quiet place for telephoning	61	56	59	55
lounge areas facing the sun	57	47	61	57
bedroom facing the sun	52	47	58	53
medibath	52	52	56	54
views of streets and roads	57	47	55	50
hallways with places for relaxing	55	47	53	50
kitchen for making tea and snacks	49	46	51	44
a low-intensity night light	43	39	45	46
moveable bedroom furniture	45	39	43	40
living in groups	38	40	38	39
a shared bedroom	27	32	30	27
provision of alcohol	37	34	25	25

Scores base = 100

communality and collective organization, such as group living and shared bedrooms, received a low priority, as did the overtly institutional medibath and the low-intensity night-light. The reasons why residents chose the 'safety against fire' card are unclear. Particular care had been taken to ensure that the card was as unemotive as possible. We can only surmise that staff anxiety concerning resident safety, the presence of heavy firedoors and other equipment, and the intense media coverage which seems to follow any fire in an old people's home, may have made an impression upon residents, who recognize their own vulnerability and dependence upon staff if such an emergency should occur.

Of course, different groups of residents ranked the cards in different ways. With increasing mental and physical frailty, residents were less likely to score highly cards which depicted aspects of environmental control such as 'easily opened windows' and were more likely to favour passive pleasures – views from windows or a lounge facing the sun. An increase in mental infirmity also led to a reduced concern for privacy, and the 'single room' card fell to an all-time low of thirty-three for the most disturbed group of residents, as opposed to a high of eighty-five for the most lucid. However, we cannot rule out the continued influence of residents' present circumstances where more confused residents are more likely to share than to occupy a single room. Increased frailty may also bring a recognition of the potential of equipment such as medibaths. In homes with a higher level of physical impairment amongst residents the score for the medibath increased, whereas the score for the ordinary bath fell. Also of particular importance with regard to the most infirm was the card depicting 'separating confused residents', the more lucid residents being much more in favour of segregation than the most frail.

While resident characteristics resulted in some variation in card rankings, aspects of the physical and social environment also made an impact. Residents living in large homes, those that were purpose built, and those which opened most recently, were more likely to rate highly features depicting environmental control and the privacy of a single room, which no doubt also reflected their current experience. In contrast, those living in older homes, often built or adapted to a more generous space standard, were more tolerant of room sharing. In terms of the social environment, a comparison of choices within group, semi-group, and non-group living homes highlights some very interesting differences. Residents in group-living homes rated more highly 'good sound insulation', 'medibaths', 'receiving friends in bedrooms', 'living in groups', and 'separating confused residents', all aspects of the environment which in some ways relate to the special nature of group-living homes. Thus 'good sound insulation' may be more important in homes where bedroom areas and sitting/dining areas are adjacent, the need for medibaths may reflect the greater physical frailty of the group home residents in our sample, and 'receiving friends in bedrooms' the desire for privacy in personal relationships advocated as part of the group system.

Our attempts in comparing the real world of residential care with residents' preferences for an ideal setting reveal two important factors. First, that even given the projective nature of the visual game, some residents still found it difficult to detach themselves from their present environment. Second, that in spite of these difficulties, residents chose many environmental features that were non-institutional and belonged to the world that they knew at home in the community. This gives some indication of the level of congruence between the needs of old people and the realities of the institutional setting. Yet, having said this, we are also aware of degrees of congruence. Although a majority of residents expressed preferences for a physical environment which offered greater privacy and environmental control, greater security in terms of a more prosthetic setting was appreciated by the more physically frail.

So, how do we marry the needs of old people for an environment over which they maintain a level of control supported by the right to privacy, continuity, and security, with the realities of institutionalization? Are some old people's homes currently providing such an environment? It would appear from our analysis that at present the answer is 'No'. While we have demonstrated that there is variation both within and between the hundred homes in terms of physical environment and organizational style, we are still left with our observations of a degree of uniformity which pervades the general atmosphere in all homes. We also accept that the variation in well-being that exists amongst elderly residents may be a function of the health, personality, and past circumstances of residents, as well as the effects of institutional living. Furthermore, by examining outcome in terms of the resident group we fail to capture the unique characteristics of individual adjustment which lie hidden in these trends. If there is to be a future for residential provision for old people then we must develop an environment that can accommodate the heterogeneity that is represented by the varying needs of residents, allowing for flexibility between autonomy and control, support and security, and enabling old people, their relatives and the residential staff, an opportunity to create an interdependent lifestyle. How this may be approached becomes the focus of our final chapters.

CHAPTER 7

Private lives in public places

We have argued that the barriers to a radical re-ordering of residential care centre around failures in the past to acknowledge the massive gulf which exists between life in the community and life in the institution. There has been an illegitimate transfer of domestic nomenclature to the institutional setting without a full appreciation of what is required to construct an authentic home environment.

We have noted and reflected the displeasure of old people who are obliged through organizational diktat to live out their individual lives in largely public and grouped settings in the residential home. There is an unreal set of expectations about what occurs when someone crosses the institutional threshold. It is assumed that new residents will discover the personal resources necessary to instigate major adjustments to a lifetime's conception of home as intimate, personal, and private in favour of a model whose physical and social dimensions are daunting and where the lifestyle is communal and public.

Residents who may be entering care to achieve a degree of support and security for their future well-being might expect to encounter a different lifestyle. But there is evidence to suggest that the strength of institutional regimes and environments goes beyond the levels of individual tolerance. In other words, at a moment in life when they experience multiple loss and start to acknowledge their own vulnerability, residents must adjust to this unique amalgam of physical strangeness, unanticipated routines, an unfamiliar peer group, and a set of formal relationships with staff – all provided in a rule-bound world.

This is the essential trait of institutional care which has not been obliterated by a catalogue of twentieth-century endeavours which are designed to erase all echoes of the past. It is these features which we can identify in all of the one hundred homes which contributed to the National Consumer Study – despite enormous variation on any one individual dimension.

It seems reasonable to suggest that our present old people's homes will retain a pejorative image as an expression of our collective concern for elderly people until we develop an alternative model for reconstructing the essence of home within an institutional framework. This in turn must be a model which will have authenticity for both residents and outsiders. And if it is to challenge that strangeness of residential care which threatens the newcomer then it must interfere in some fundamental way with environmental attributes which deny personal history and integrity and individual freedoms; it must be designed to promote the enjoyment of private lives in public places.

Restructuring the environment

In order to reverse those features of residential life which impose a block against expressions of individuality on the part of residents, it becomes necessary to question the basic unit of operation around which the activities of daily living are programmed. Inevitably, we are forced to conclude that for most purposes and in most places the size of the unit is equal to the total population of the home.

Evidence to support this statement is provided by a number of institutional 'props': for example, most homes will have a bath-book which locates various individuals against time slots available as bath-times and personnel available as bath aides – the detailed construction of individual care programmes showing that Mrs Jones likes to be bathed before her visitors arrive on Saturdays and Sundays, in the morning, and preferably by care assistants A or D, is notable by its common absence. Similar evidence might be cited in relation to mid-morning coffee breaks – served in the dining-room only, to residents but not to their visitors, between 10.45 and 11.00 a.m., irrespective of the fact that Mr Smith is very concerned by his sister's infrequent visits and is reluctant to leave her to get coffee for himself alone, thus disrupting their difficult, personal exchange.

A cursory glance at the routines of a residential home will confirm that the old people as individuals *qua* individuals have ceased to exist. They do not represent the basic unit of operation around which residential life is constructed. The organization is predicated around a group logic.

Over a period of time there has undoubtedly been a reduction in the size of the unit insofar as establishments have come to accommodate fewer residents. Since the turn of the century, average size has reduced from one hundred or more to a mere forty today. Furthermore, the introduction of group living has ostensibly reduced the unit size from around numbers of between forty and fifty to groups of eight or ten. But the important point demonstrated by the National Consumer Study findings is that routinized treatment of residents can persist across all of these changes in scale and changes in type, so that an individual elderly person simply cannot maintain personal integrity and self-esteem in the face of this set of institutional forces.

Indeed, we would question the logic which suggests that a group of eight or ten is deemed to be closer to the individual old person than a group of forty, for it is undoubtedly the case that throughout their lives people live as members of families or as single people; their intimate and domestic moments are not generally shared with groups of any size. For a wealthy minority, a public school upbringing might lurk in their distant past and, for men, the enforced camaraderie of the armed services might serve as a role model. But there has never been any hint that, for the majority, communal living could build on earlier experience.

It does not follow, then, that small group living for the elderly can deal with this problem of the unit of operation, for, while small group living legitimately aims to scale down the physical and organizational forms of residential living, the aim to create a surrogate family setting must be regarded as illegitimate. The intimacies of blood relationship cannot be foisted upon the artificial grouping devised for group living; the alternative relationships which skilled social work interventions may produce are at best an amelioration of mass living over which limited control can be extended by group members.

Sadly, at an empirical level, we can demonstrate that in institutions where group living operates, the influence of the larger establishment can negate any benefit which might be attributed to the organizational strategy of group living. Hence there remains a continuing need to devise ways of making the individual old person the basic and unique building block of the residential establishment.

Developing a new philosophy in care

Much of the evidence that has been presented in this text confirms the view that an adequate rationale for residential care has never been fully developed. The definition in the National Assistance Act, 1948, provides us with a necessary but insufficient explanation for a policy which aims to deliver care in an institutional setting rather than in the community. In a sense, there is a deliberate attempt to offer something that is distinct and separate from the familiar mix of domiciliary support services; yet the explanation for this sharp dichotomy cannot be traced in the policy document and there is a blurring of the process which might direct a client along route A or route B.

Reordering the residential environment might usefully start with a dramatic challenge to this instance of separation and develop an argument for services to be managed in such a way that residential care can move back into the embrace of the community in which it is located. Hence, the residential alternative would become just one more point along the increasingly sensitive spectrum of community care options.

We have noted earlier the historical tendency of policy-makers to retain at their disposal the institutional solution 'pour encourager les autres'; that is, it was a powerful deterrent to that deviant group of workshy and feckless old persons whose lifetime of irresponsibility had brought them to impecunity. The inappropriateness of this analysis is self-evident in a welfare state which, despite shifts in economic policy, has not yet fully reneged on a promise of care and support from the cradle to the grave. And to reverse these negative images it becomes necessary to reorder and relocate residential services so that they represent an attractive alternative to the best that is on offer within community care.

This in turn implies a massive programme of what is commonly referred to as 'normalization'. This seemingly grand title describes a process whose success lies in its stark simplicity. One definition refers to:

> 'The use of means which are valued in our society in order to develop and support personal behaviour experiences and characteristics: which are likewise valued.'
>
> (Campaign for Mentally Handicapped People 1981: 1)

The aim would be to devise a form of care that old people and their carers might choose on the basis of the particular balance of security and freedoms that can be achieved in a residential setting. This involves three sets of assumptions: first, that responsible authorities will have a view to the heterogeneity of the population they are serving and develop, accordingly, services that are different in kind but equivalent in status for different needs and different aspirations; second, that sufficient information will be provided to clients in a manner that enables them to negotiate the optimum package of care for their personal requirements after weighing up the 'gains' and 'losses' inherent in the various options; and third, that old people will be encouraged and assisted to work their way through this gains and losses equation so that they are in a position to exercise real consumer choice.

The new philosophy of care emerging from such developments becomes one in which a secure environment is offered to the frail, and perhaps fearful, old person who selects this residential option. It is one which insulates the client from some of the more onerous aspects of living in the community but does not isolate him or her from a previous world in which freedom of choice and familiarity are taken-for-granted elements.

Shifts will inevitably occur in the transition from natural home to residential home but they should represent a shift in degree, not in kind, for it must be assumed that the freedoms of a perhaps housebound person are already delimited by the physical structures of his or her home and a reduced circle of callers; choice is restricted to what can be achieved indoors; and familiarity will focus on friends and the domestic setting; already the familiarity of well-known streets, shops, and neighbourhood visits will have had to be given up. In the residential home a different set of limitations will come into play but the aim of residential carers, together with clients, must be to push the boundaries of 'normalization' to their furthest limits.

One obvious starting-point for attempting to redress the balance of residential living is the point at which the individual resident loses control in an environment which, while it has been designed to offer shelter and protected home territory, in fact often represents an extremely impoverished socio-spatial world, where choice and control are virtually non-existent. Thus we would aim to restore residents' opportunity to exercise environmental control while maintaining necessary levels of physical and social support.

We start, then, from the clients' needs as they emerge from the National Consumer Study – their desire to achieve the normal, the unexceptional, and the non-institutional. This is a set of demands which is coloured by differences of emphasis amongst different members of the resident population yet represent in some form a common aspiration for all groups. Meeting these demands would mean constructing a framework within which elderly people might use their own material and metaphysical resources to create a new home, and we might anticipate that the residents' ideal home will not necessarily reproduce an image of home life which corresponds with that of the residential 'professionals'.

Taking our cue from the choices made by old people, we must begin by identifying those features of existing arrangements which threaten their ability to achieve dignity and self-esteem. At a macro level we would wish to demonstrate explicitly to our clients and to those who care about their well-being that we are prepared to construct environments that are a worthy setting for our respected elders. We must assert, by the nature of the old age home, that it offers a meaningful life for people who are valued and cherished. To be more specific, this will mean a comprehensive assault to challenge and obliterate the deep offence caused by characteristics such as institutional smell, institutional noise, and institutional infantilization of old people.

At a pragmatic level and as a crucial tool for implementing policy change, we are talking about the development of a care-providers' checklist (Kellaher, Peace and Willocks 1985) to the world of care. This would highlight pathways to good practice through a series of crucial do's and don'ts addressed to all those whose work touches upon residential care. At the current stage of shifting to a new philosophy of care this must be regarded as a necessary tactical device to prompt institutional change.

At a more fundamental level, however, we must prepare a rigorous strategy for challenging the social and physical construction of residential care around the assumption that old people will be prepared, in the role of residents, to live out their remaining years in largely public settings in the home. What follows is that they do not have proper access to private space and the major part of their waking hours must be spent in the company of others. This accords with organizational imperatives for managing old age homes and it facilitates the efficient undertaking of staff 'surveillance' duties. This represents part of the care task which is more confidently carried out when residents are assembled collectively, in limited space, rather than dispersed throughout the institution.

A strategy for reversing this emphasis demands that the focus of the home switches from public living in communal space to private living in personal space. Under such arrangements the unit of operation for organizational purposes would be the individual resident; hence the needs of the individual would take precedence as a means of serving the group, and any block treatment would be rendered unacceptable. And, returning briefly to the notion of a care-providers' checklist, it would be quite unthinkable, when planning an individual care programme for Mrs Jones, to expect her to function in accordance with her own wishes, habits, and standards in personal space, yet in the public area be exposed to the clatter of traditional institutional dining arrangements, the smell of last night's meal or worse, and the generalized demeaning label of 'gran'. If private living-in personal space is taken seriously, then it must have inevitable spill-over effects for the activities that take place on common ground. The demands of residents, once realized, for an ordinary way of life, will not be confined to private territory; they will extend to lounges, dining-rooms, and bathing areas with the dramatic effect of revitalizing the very foundations of institutional care.

How is this to be achieved? In order to implement change of this magnitude it is argued that the following broad shifts in care patterns are necessary: a transformation of spatial arrangements between public and private space; a positive reorientation of the relationship between the old age home and the wider community; and the introduction of practical support for a new philosophy in residential living, that is organizational change based on substantially revised staff-training programmes.

The transformation of spatial arrangements suggests a process that is instigated at the drawing-board, that is it implies substantial physical reorganization that is best introduced through the design of a new residential home or major adaptation to an existing home. Certainly this provides the most fortuitous set of circumstances for remodelling care patterns and, for any local authorities who may have succeeded in protecting their capital programme for new-build and renewal from externally imposed financial restraint, this offers one major avenue for implementation. In this context, architects would be encouraged to enhance the status of private territory by making individual residents' rooms the focus of personal territory. At the same time, evidence suggests that greater proximity between private and public space will encourage a more natural relationship between the two parts of the home; routes that are designed to facilitate this integration can assist the frail resident to manage and control the physical environment. In homes where the potential for capital involvement is limited, then attention will switch to physical accoutrements and organizational devices that serve the same ends.

In practice this might mean the introduction of an area for relaxation and friendly exchanges located within a bedroom wing that is separated from the main living area. This could be achieved by adaptations such as using excess hallway space for locating armchairs plus a coffee table, or by a change of use of a bedroom to sitting space. Where bedrooms are too small for additional personal furniture, it is possible to experiment with properly located wall furniture in order to have a colourful mix of personal items. Where bedrooms must be shared it is possible to divide areas using screening, which can also be used to affix pot plants, pictures, or craft items. And, where corridors appear institutional and daunting under the glare of strip lighting reflecting on plastic floors, the introduction of appropriate carpet tiles together with supplementary soft wall lights can make a lengthy journey less onerous. An inventory of innovative and cost-effective devices might readily be developed to shift the ethos of the physical world and thereby produce a less alien environment to those unaccustomed to institutional settings.

The second part of the strategy would be to take advantage of the improved image of the home and use this as a base upon which to build a more positive and productive relationship between the home and the community in which it is located. If the home appears less threatening to outsiders, then the trauma of transition will be dramatically reduced; moreover, the possibility of residents making real relationships with people and places around their former home is increased if the psychological distance involved in the move has been likewise reduced.

One of the ways in which the outsider's fear of institutional settings can be alleviated is by optimizing the capital and revenue resources used in running a home and, with appropriate safeguards for residents, opening up the facilities and providing services to other members of the community; short-stay or respite care together with day care are two possibilities which can extend the boundaries of the old age home. And where the home forms a normal and unexceptional part of that community's spectrum of care options then mutual benefits can accrue to both resident and occasional home user. But there are serious issues around residents' rights and the defence of home territory.

This raises the question of how this reordering of residential care is going to be implemented on a day-to-day basis – where the same level of demand for care and support will be expressed by the same group of frail and vulnerable residents to the same group of staff. We have shown that staff members already experience the care task as comprising an unceasing stream of tiring and time-consuming activities in which physical care and domestic duties around the needs of residents exhaust all available time.

The simple answer is that the care task must be developed into an alternative form of care, and heads of homes together with their care staff will require an investment of appropriate resources to make this transition feasible. Proper training facilities will be required to inculcate a new approach to the care task, thereby shifting attitudes to give priority to facilitating rather than doing, and to social and emotional care in favour of elements of detail contained within the domestic round. Open discussion of difficult issues like the right to risk will allow staff the opportunity to express their anxieties; proper support from senior management on policies that encourage residents to control key aspects of their own lives will be a crucial part of developing resident freedoms and the possibility of retaining a private life within the residential setting.

The residential flatlet

There are undoubtedly several ways in which the normalization of residential establishments can be attempted through shifts in design and organization. We have charted earlier a number of residential fashions which have influenced the nature of care and caring; all have stimulated amelioration yet none has been grounded in a rigorous analysis of the relationship between institutions and communities. Arguably, therefore, they have failed to achieve 'breakthrough' in reconstituting residential care with the exception perhaps of Lipman and Slater (1977a), who have produced sensitive design solutions.

The arguments that have been developed from our analysis of evidence emerging from the National Consumer Study do present a more fundamental reappraisal of the process of care provision and care delivery. This is a necessary function of acknowledging the legitimacy and authenticity of the consumers' voice. When residents opted for the normal, the unexceptional, and the non-institutional they would often challenge the conventional wisdom of policy-makers, choosing a lifestyle that reflects as far as possible the everyday taken-for-granted aspects of living in the community.

Accordingly a specific model of care has been constructed from their statements which attempts to articulate consumer aspirations. It is not envisaged that this model will meet the demands for all possible worlds by all possible residents, but it reflects a flexible option that can develop the contours of care in ways that extend consumer choice and control. The focus for change suggested by the National Consumer Study is the establishment of a facility termed the residential flatlet (*Figure 9*).

This would be the point of entry and stability within the institution for an individual old person coming into care. It would constitute a larger and more flexible version of the existing single room, different from sheltered housing insofar as it would remain part of an essentially supportive environment. Yet the residential flatlet would offer unmistakeable personal territory, lockable from the inside, and within it the resident would be firmly in control of everyday routine. The nature of the shift from community life to living in care would thus change radically since occupancy of this type of facility would enable entry to a residential establishment to occur in a way which corresponds to

Figure 9 Residential flatlet

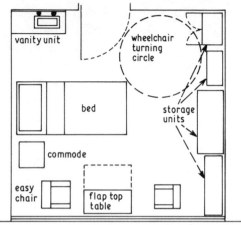

sketch layout of resident's living room (15 m² approx.)

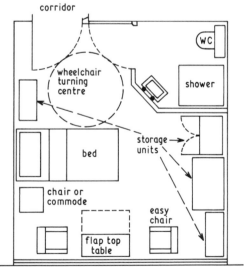

sketch layout of resident's living-room with shower room
and WC en suite (18 m² approx.)

'moving house' rather than surrendering to some admissions process imposed from outside by other people. So the old person might anticipate relocating his or her home as opposed to leaving home.

This flatlet should be large enough to accommodate some personal items of substantial furniture such as a bed or a sideboard which might evoke significant memories and affirm individual status and identity. Sufficient space must be allowed for residents to sit in comfort alone or with their visitors. Tea-making equipment would be provided. It is not envisaged that this room would contain elaborate cooking facilities; main catering would be undertaken centrally but meals could be taken and shared with neighbours or visitors in the individual flatlets.

In order to preserve and protect those areas of independence appropriate to and achievable by different residents, a range of support services would then be built around the flatlet: sanitary services such as a vanity unit would form an integral part of the flatlet, or be located adjacent to it, as would the shower plus WC. Baths would be provided separately. Two levels of catering would be necessary to offer centrally prepared and served meals for those who chose to be served, and self-catering in a kitchenette for those who chose to help themselves. Residents and visitors might then make snacks or prepare a light breakfast and share their food in accordance with the normal social mores of entertaining and visiting. At least one large lounge must also be offered, possibly incorporating part of the entrance hall, as an alternative meeting-place. An additional focal point would avoid potential problems of residents becoming isolated in their rooms – particularly the more frail and immobile.

In order to facilitate free movement around the residential establishment it is necessary to ensure that public and private domains be clearly distinguished, but separation must not be such that movement between the two areas becomes difficult or hazardous. In addition, homes must be designed to incorporate key features which promote familiarity and trigger orientation within the macro-environment. Basic design features should assist residents to recognize the shape of the whole building, thus rendering the physical world comprehensible. These broad changes in physical design are recommended to stimulate an alternative lifestyle which permits old people to recreate the essential features contained within their idea of home – on private territory, in personal space.

Quality of home life

It is argued that the possibility of preserving a private life in the residential setting will be advantageous to old people in a number of ways. We have shown that residents in general do aspire towards self-determination in the ordinary activities of daily living. The kind of environmental decision-making that was generated by the visual game in the National Consumer Study reflects a consistent desire to control the physical and social world of care. Within the context of the residential flatlet such opportunities will be more likely to develop.

A particular instance of the importance of environmental control occurs in relation to gender difference. Information gathered for the National Consumer Study demonstrated that in many ways the residential process may prove a qualititatively different kind of experience for men and for women. Women tend to enter care at a later point in the ageing process, and for different reasons from men; as a consequence, problems of adjustment may prove more onerous for them. They tend to be more frail at the point of entry; many more women were previously living alone, in circumstances where they could control their lives, and it tended to be a general physical deterioration and inability to cope which precipitated admission. Thus, unlike their younger and fitter male counterparts, women in traditional old age homes appear less able to 'control' their daily routine in terms of moving around the building and participating in a range of interesting activities, either of a recreational or domestic character.

The quality of new social relationships developed in institutions may not adequately meet women's needs for friendship, and the nature of the constrained residential visit may not prove conducive to the continuation of intimate relationships with outside family or friends. Living in small groups may offer the promise of a different lifestyle imbued with activity and meaning, but in practice this promise may fail to materialize where organizational constraints at the level of the whole establishment inhibit the creation of dynamic and coherent group structures.

One means of improving life quality for women residents would be to offer practical compensation for problems resulting from 'loss of home' and the threat to their traditional domestic and nurturing role.

This might be achieved through the more individual lifestyle which is associated with the residential flatlet. In the privacy of personal territory it becomes possible to express important aspects of self-identity using treasured mementoes from earlier in life. Evidence points to an increase in the rate of new friendship formation and adjustment to the positive possibilities of residential living amongst those who achieve such personal autonomy and environmental control.

We have argued that, in order for life in the residential home to present a popular appeal to old people presently located in the community, there must be a strengthening of links between the home and the community. This in turn would enhance the quality of life for those presently resident insofar as the diminishing of institutional atmosphere through the delineation of personal territory would provide the framework for a rich and varied social life which is not delimited by the walls of the institution. For a home built upon individual flatlets represents a more attractive and structured environment for outsiders coming in and the socio-spatial arrangements inside the home would encourage social interaction in real space, either for individual exchanges or for group activity. Furthermore, this degree of normality would support the expectation of residents that service-providers with whom they have developed relationships in the community, be they social workers, district nurses, or GPs, should cross the threshold and extend their services inside the world of residential care.

This in turn prompts consideration of the situation that will arise when the facilities of a residential establishment are shared by those with a permanent entitlement to residence and those with the status of day attender or short-stay resident. Evidence from traditional homes suggests that conflict can often arise among different users when the institutional expectations of persons who are resident appear to be threatened by a group of strangers. In contrast, the way in which public and private space becomes divided in the context of residential flatlets could ensure that residents' rights are not violated by others who might seek to extend the activities of the home beyond those of simply providing long-term care.

In the past, opposing demands and expectations between residents and others have, in some instances, had a detrimental effect on social relationships in the home. Day attenders might look at the frailty and apathy of residents and experience real fears for their own future yet, at the same time, they may feel envy for the security and service that accompany residential living as compared with the difficulties they may experience in the community; therefore, they may make heavy demands on staff time while they are in the home. The other side of the coin is that residents may perceive day attenders or short-stay residents as intruders and this might cause them to resent the encroachment on scarce staffing resources.

Individual residential flatlet accommodation would, in contrast, change, in a positive direction, the image of residents as real people for outsiders coming in, and it would help to allay their anxieties; the provision of personal lockable space would offer a material framework for residents' rights, and it might then be possible for residents and day attenders to forge mutually satisfying social relationships as comparative equals. Staff care time could then be allocated more effectively to the different requirements of each group.

Similar advantages to residents and outsiders might accrue in relation to short-stay beds, either for assessment purposes or for respite care. Residential flatlets offer a less all-consuming model for experiencing institutional care. For old people relocated to a residential home for a temporary period only, this would alleviate the strangeness of a new environment; it would reduce the more disruptive effects of being moved and enable residential care staff and residents alike to receive the newcomers as welcome guests. Recent research has shown that under current arrangements this combined service can produce major problems, both for staff and the different user groups (Allen 1983).

It is argued, then, that the promotion of community integration is a natural corollary of a restructured lifestyle which emphasizes the benefits of leading a private life in a public institution. This new model would attract more outsiders into the home and thereby make life more vital and real inside the residential establishment; this in turn would generate increased interest and opportunities for residents to venture outside the home for social visiting and seeking out familiar places. The reordering of internal arrangements would provide a vehicle for challenging all those aspects of residential life which suggest a total institution, and it would enable staff and residents to share together in a vigorous campaign to establish the home and its people within the mainstream of community life.

Quality of working life

It has been emphasized that residents need to achieve a degree of self-determination or 'mastery' in the ordinary taken-for-granted activities of daily life (Clough 1981). Yet under present institutional arrangements there is an implicit organizational commitment to a form of task allocation which promotes staff surveillance and the avoidance of risk-taking. This elimination of the rights to engage in normal, but low-risk, activities threatens the ability of old people in care settings to achieve some degree of independence and live a life away from the public gaze of anxious care staff.

Moreover, this represents the inherent conflict of interests which arises when the same establishment must be designed and managed as an appropriate home environment for one group of users and an adequate work environment for another group. Residents look for an environment designed to offer maximum flexibility, continuity, and real friendship from their carers – and packages of care delivered at a pace and with a demeanour that respects both the frailty and the importance of the client. Residential staff, in contrast, generally require a routine bounded by a set of rules together with a predetermined set of responsibilities that is strictly timetabled to allow them to complete their busy daily round.

It seems likely that the structure offered by residential flatlets would permit residents and staff to counteract this dilemma and try to resolve the difficult question of promoting resident choice and freedom while simultaneously providing staff with an adequate rationale and appropriate supports for redefining the care task. Under present institutional arrangements, a major part of staff time is taken up with the performance of physical care tasks. Little time is available to develop the role of facilitator or to enable residents to help themselves and it is unusual for staff to allocate specific time for meeting the social needs of residents. Indeed there is confusion regarding the extent to which staff members should engage in social exchanges with their clients. An experiment with the use of residential volunteers (Power *et al.*

1984) demonstrated initial common agreement amongst all parties that it would be the role of volunteers to strike up new friendships with clients while care staff were free to pursue the important duties like physical care and tending. Yet it was ultimately found to be more advantageous to the resident when these roles of volunteer and statutory carer were reversed, for what the residents required was the continuity and reliability of real social exchanges with people who are seen not just for the occasional hour or two every week, but across the whole week.

The residential flatlet could be regarded as the physical prompt for massive shifts in defining the residential care task. This would be to the advantage of worker and resident alike. A prerequisite for essential shifts might be the routine introduction of a key worker scheme which aimed to restore the resident's confidence and thereby introduced the real possibility of an increase in resident mastery; at the same time, care would be construed as relating to individual need rather than a set of global demands presented by the resident population as a whole.

Such an approach provides a focus for replacing what might be regarded as maternalistic or disabling practices in favour of a more enabling style of care. This is not to suggest that the physical care of dependent persons together with domestic chores would disappear; residents could be encouraged to retain domestic and self-care skills where this was realistic but inevitably staff would continue to bear the major responsibility within these areas. Nevertheless it is suggested that this broadening of the concept of care would ultimately prove beneficial to staff. Moreover, this question of care priorities, leading to a revised conception of the care task, could offer a better basis for designing long-overdue staff-training packages for care assistants.

Perhaps one of the most frustrating difficulties for the residential sector is the experience of having to respond to shifts elsewhere in the support network at a time when demographic change will ensure an increase in overall numbers of the very old and frail. First, there has been a dramatic decline in the number of long-stay geriatric beds and district health authorities have launched a vigorous assault on those whom they label 'geriatric bedblockers' with a view to securing a more efficient use of NHS resources. A second factor relates to the reduced capacity of the community to provide informal support as a consequence of the migration of the caring family and the increased involvement of women carers in the world of work. Third, a pro rata decrease in domiciliary support services compounds the difficulties experienced by old people living alone. One further influence may be exerted by the dramatic extension of private residential homes in the care network. The fear has been expressed that they may be selective in offering care to a fitter and less demanding group among the potential clientele.

The net result is a complex set of pressures on residential places. This may result in allocation policies which favour the construction of a more dependent clientele for Part III in terms of levels of frailty and confusion. Some evidence (Charlesworth and Wilkin 1982) suggests that this may not be as globally extensive as earlier commentators feared, but the question this raises is how may staff best cope when the levels of dependency fluctuate over comparatively short periods of time within a given establishment.

Some writers argue that good practice can be created for the most frail in a specialist environment. There is another view which has persisted over time which favours integration (MIND 1979; Evans *et al.* 1981). Arguably, where proper resources are provided for both staff and residents, a non-specialist home can tolerate substantial proportions of confused and physically frail residents. And it is possible that the routine introduction of the specialist home as a discrete option along the care continuum (from minimum support to twenty-four-hour nursing care) may produce one further stage in the discontinuity of care, with elderly people being subjected, as their needs change, to a series of disruptive and largely unsolicited moves through the care system.

An establishment where territory is divided more clearly into public and private spaces and constructed around individual flatlets would assist staff who are dealing with a mix of dependency levels. It would be possible to develop personalized packages of care and deliver them individually in ways which essentially protect the interests of the 'fit' from those of the 'unfit' and vice versa, while securing a fair deal for both groups individually and reducing conflict between them. For example, the privacy of a single bedsitting room permits adaptation around the special needs of the individual client together with the creation of a personalized environment which can be imbued with history and meaning, thereby assisting the frail confused to retain or reinforce existing skills and orientation. And this can provide an alternative strategy for dealing with the more 'difficult' resident. There is increasing evidence to suggest (Wade *et al*. 1983) that an excessive use of drug therapy has become the norm in some homes and that this is associated with behavioural difficulties. It becomes an urgent matter to explore alternative environmental strategies as a means of reversing this trend.

Conclusions

The substance of this chapter has been to explore the broad issues around privacy and normal living in an institutional setting by abstracting data from the National Consumer Study to show that the ability to control physical and metaphysical space is a key factor in enabling the elderly person to enter residential care without losing the ability to live an independent and fulfilling life. Essentially this means that we must respond, in policy terms, to the needs of individuals to protect their personal space from the threat of institutional invasion if we are serious in our stated intention to protect and preserve the rights of residents to be themselves and to live their own lives.

It has been possible to indicate in earlier chapters the nature of the reciprocal relationship between institutional design and institutional organization. The way in which physical territory is structured has a powerful impact on the way in which the occupants of that territory – residents and workers alike – order their daily round. Clustered lavatories and bathrooms located some distance away from a resident's bedroom ensure that the use of these facilities is rendered institutional in appearance and in use, and they exist beyond the physical and mental space which the resident feels able to control. Bedrooms of an inadequate size, where furniture and fittings are permanently affixed, tend to offer minimum scope for personalization and work against the creation of a homelike dwelling for retreat and relaxation.

Equally, the careful structuring of the residential day in accordance with a strict timetable, where dull but persistent routine is punctuated by the flurry of activity around institutional meal-times, has a profound impact on the way in which different parts of the home are used. Staffing arrangements produce regimes which limit the possibility of developing work patterns that are resident oriented as opposed to institution oriented.

In seeking to construct a residential alternative, the determining factor for us has been to identify ways of challenging this status quo. It is crucially important that the conflict between different interest groups in the home should be addressed explicitly and that any proposal for institutional change serves as a device for supporting the vulnerable old person in his or her inevitable struggle against the power of the mass institution. At the same time, the interests of dedicated staff must be respected.

The residential flatlet that we have described offers one such avenue for change. Not only does the physical world of the individual accord with a situation in which this relatively small room can, literally, shut out unwelcome institutional messages but also it provides a power base which enables the resident to develop constructive survival strategies for coping more effectively when he or she does enter the public arena. And it has been argued that, where public and private space are clearly delineated, the net result is a powerful shift of emphasis among both spectators and collaborators – the world on the outside of residential care and the staff on the inside – so that attention always turns away from the prospect of mass living and towards the positive reconstruction of private and personal lives in these public places.

CHAPTER 8

Unfinished business

The essence of this text has been to reveal the limits of residential living. We have charted institutional developments over one and a half centuries and produced a critique of present services. Much of the evidence from a study of one hundred homes points to the enormous strides that have been made in residential services. This can be measured in terms of dramatic changes which are visible in both physical and organizational dimensions of residential settings. But at the same time we have been obliged to confront divergences between the aspirations of stated policy and observed residential practice. While the public appearances of people and places may change it is quite apparent that private attitudes towards them may lag. There is much to suggest that society at large fails to acknowledge that it is a positive achievement to enable more people to survive into old age, a tribute to improved public health and welfare provision. Instead, we observe a rolling back of the welfare state as part of an explicit policy switch in which social policy and the needs of vulnerable groups become subordinate to economism. This in turn generates a fear that non-productive individuals may prove an onerous charge on dwindling resources, and there is a grudging policy response which, in the case of old people, is translated through and focused upon the form of the old age home.

It is the purpose of this chapter to enquire whether the residential professionals have given up their attempts to make a positive contribution to the welfare of old people by creating appropriate residential environments. Is the evidence against institutions so overwhelming that society should abandon attempts to promote change or are there clues within this account of residential life which might direct us to a potentially successful alternative to present arrangements?

We have shown that cosmetic changes in built form or care routines constitute a necessary but insufficient impetus to real change. Their impact is negated by an uncaring world which tends to marginalize old people and which imposes arbitrary limits on attempts at institutional reform. Time and time again innovative schemes have been introduced with a fanfare of optimism, as in the case of group living, only to be infiltrated by traditional mores in the face of societal indifference. What we have shown is that it is not possible to carry through the full implications of such reforms in the absence of a fundamental challenge to the attitudes of those who run the residential services; this in turn must be associated with substantial shifts in the way society as a whole values its older members.

We have argued that one way in which this challenge might be taken up and sustained is through the concept of 'normalization'. In other words, the care relationships and institutional arrangements in which a group of people like the elderly become involved as clients, must be designed to assert and confirm primary societal values. In this way, the rights of older people to make choices and achieve dignity become paramount.

However, we have witnessed and recorded, through a catalogue of residential misdemeanours and inappropriate treatments, a deep-rooted persistence of what is, at its worst, large-scale dehumanization of clients, and at best a redefinition and a narrowing of human potential. The central argument that we have developed as an approach to reversing this negative form of residential process is that providing personal territory offers the possibility of preserving an individual and private lifestyle. What remains unclear at this moment in welfare history is whether this strategy will have sufficient force to combat the magnitude of institutional oppression that has defeated the best efforts of generations of social reformers.

Current issues

It is generally agreed that change in residential care is long overdue. Moreover, there are immediate issues arising from recent changes in social structure which are reinforced by the restructuring of welfare – a phenomenon that has achieved some degree of sophistication as a direct result of government policy. Accordingly it is appropriate in this final chapter to examine a series of current developments: shifts in public-sector care and the dramatic growth of private old people's homes; the debate about the significance of institutional built form; feminist arguments for the rights of women to control their own lives which are coupled with the demand for adequate and appropriate statutory care services for dependent relatives; the growing recognition of demands from ethnic minority groups for services that will meet the needs of a new generation of ethnic elders; and the struggle between central government and the local state, as attempts to control the public purse place enormous pressures on local government officials. At the same time we should also explore the welcome creation of progressive local policies – developed in hard times – and ask how they might contribute to a revitalized public-sector residential service.

Private residential care

Over the past five years the debate on residential care has been thrown into some confusion by the sudden growth in the private sector. There is evidence that government is seeking to persuade local authorities that it would be beneficial to develop innovative forms of community care that could capitalize on the contribution of informal carers. At the same time, incentives have been provided for an initially small, but resilient, private residential sector to expand at what has turned out to be an exponential rate. In 1979 there were 15,000 beds in private rest homes, and in just four years that has quadrupled to 60,000 beds.

While this is not the arena to debate the advantages and disadvantages of private social care, it is important to highlight the implications of recent changes in the balance of care for the future of residential services. The questions this poses, at the level of the individual, relate to consumer choice and control. If elderly people are prepared to go out and buy private care in the market-place does this mean that professionals have been unduly hasty in mobilizing support for alternatives to residential care? There are questions raised concerning the level of community responsibility for developing appropriate services which will meet consumer demands. The sudden surge of private care threatens the ability of democratically elected authorities to plan services in relation to need and to achieve service goals of allocative efficiency and distributive justice.

However, this gives us pause to reflect on present inadequacies in public services and the manner in which some paying customers can obtain a service through the market-place. When old people buy care they experience some degree of choice and control over their destiny in old age. What concerns some observers (Vladeck 1980) is the possibility that the production of care for profit may lead to practices which are the antithesis of normalization in terms of lifestyle at home.

Furthermore, there is the possibility that dependency levels in public and private sectors may be distorted by different modes of entry into care and the absence of formal assessment in the private sector. In terms of the debate on residential futures, then, it might benefit the statutory carer to enquire what characteristics in the private home attract the paying customer and how these might be replicated within the local authority service. At the same time, it will be important for local authorities to respond positively to their increased responsibilities for the regulation of private care (Weaver, Willcocks, and Kellaher 1985) and to introduce the kind of inspection and monitoring system that will protect clients from any possible abuse.

The feminist case for retaining residential homes

While social commentators have on many occasions, quite legitimately, produced devastating critiques of residential services – and in some cases (Townsend 1981) argued for their abolition – they have rarely traced the present community alternative to its logical conclusion which generally ends up with elderly daughters looking after mothers, or older women looking after their older menfolk. A recent article has taken us to task on this account (Finch 1984) and the author produces a case for revitalizing, and if necessary extending, residential provision as a means of releasing daughters, or indeed wives of dependent husbands, from the burden of care which society has imposed upon them. The argument hinges on the need for society to accept a collective responsibility for the well-being of dependent people needing care. This would restore freedom to the individual carer, who is generally a woman, and enable her to pursue her own life, or in many cases to opt for shared care.

The emphasis of government is that community carers should bear the main responsibility for looking after the increasing number of frail elderly people. This moral obligation is presented against a backcloth of demographic change which substantially affects family structure. There is the increasing divorce rate leading to more complex family patterns, the increasing proportion of women both choosing to and obliged to work outside the home, and there is presently a greater geographical separation amongst families. The myth that families do not care for their dependent members has now been demolished (Shanas 1979); successive reports show that they do so, and often at enormous cost to themselves. Perhaps one of the greatest problems experienced by these predominantly female carers is that the services which they do provide are invisible – until such time as they break down. Often it is only when a crisis occurs and someone comes along from the Town Hall to pick up the human pieces that the work of carers receives due acknowledgement.

It is a self-evident, just, and reasonable claim that is made on behalf of the carers that society should share in the important task of providing for its senior citizens. To the extent that such provision respects the rights and freedoms of those citizens to live in environments which reflect the worth and importance of the residents, then there would appear to be common cause between those who argue for a proper residential option from the feminist corner and those who argue from a socio-environmental position. However, the views of these older, and mainly female, recipients of care are also pertinent here. All turns on the adequacy of the particular residential option and the capacity of the kind of substantial shifts outlined above to construct an attractive residential life that old people will want to choose.

Providing services for ethnic minority elders

One of the dilemmas facing service-providers in the inner city is the need to cater adequately for a new generation of old people from ethnic minority communities, predominantly of Afro-Caribbean or Asian origin who have raised families and grown old in this country. At the present time they do not figure prominently as clients of statutory services, and this raises the possibility that they may suffer discrimination on the basis of both age and ethnicity. It is not clear whether they have chosen not to enter local authority homes or whether they have been obliged to refuse a place that has failed to take account of those special needs which arise out of religious or cultural differences.

If proper choice is to be the paramount consideration in providing services for all clients, then it will be necessary to deal positively with those features of present arrangements which deter the black or Asian client. Recent research (Norman 1985) points to the inappropriateness of traditional myths about black people such as 'they prefer to be with their own kind'. Changes in family structure which limit the capacity for family support highlight the need for a further investigation of the phenomenon of low take-up. There is a possibility that discrimination experienced earlier in life may discourage a person in old age from seeking new forms of help for fear of further rejection.

Yet residential homes, as environments which can be 'controlled', offer the potential for dealing specifically with complex cultural issues involving food, language, and religion – either through local authority provision or by means of support for self-help community projects, designed around local needs. The guiding principle for developing good practice must rest upon a balance between a positive recognition of cultural and racial differences which informs, but does not prejudice, assessment decision. It seems likely that a reconstruction of residential care where territory and lifestyle assume priority would offer the best way forward for meeting the particular needs of these groups of old people.

Struggles between central government and the local state

Over recent years, as the monetarist philosophy has developed into a hard-edged tool of government, there has been a persistent tension over control of the public purse as central government departments have tried to encourage local authorities towards greater thrift and prudence. This has occurred at a time when local authority departments have experienced increased demands from communities across a range of strategic support services. Ultimately it is likely to be the client who gets trapped within this wedge – and since elderly people form a substantial and increasing proportion of the client group they will suffer disproportionately.

What this means is that the reduction of rate support grant to local authorities has an immediate influence on the numbers employed in a given service – and there will be a tendency to economize by reducing revenue costs on those services which can be marginalized in some way. Capital investment in bricks and mortar will tend to be protected; moreover, the staffing of institutions cannot be reduced beyond certain negotiated levels. Hence there is likely to be a reduction in community services before the residential home is substantially affected. There is an argument, therefore, that if service-providers turn their attention to ways of developing residential care as part of an integrated package of community care, then they are more likely to preserve the best of a range of options for the greatest number of old people.

Developing progressive service alternatives

In recent years, many local authorities have undergone a period of demoralization which can be attributed to a combination of frustration at the level of government intervention in the way they run their services, together with deep anxiety at the level of service that they can continue to offer. Nevertheless, many of them have succeeded in attempts to develop models of progressive practice which start to open up the possibility for effecting real change. The form in which those initiatives may emerge will vary from locality to locality and it is likely that some will incorporate residential living and some will not. But what links a number of these schemes, which have all appeared in times of economic and social duress, is that they are firmly rooted in the local democratic process; as a result, they all take on aspects of the character of the particular area in which they have been generated. So Sheffield has produced the concept of the Elderly Persons Support Unit (MacDonald, Qureshi, and Walker 1984) where a range of social support needs for a geographically defined population of elderly people is met by workers located in one central building linked closely with community volunteers working in and around the same neighbourhood. The Isle of Wight has turned the image of a day centre on its head by designing a residential club for elderly people, where the ethos and the activities attract a wide range of individuals for recreation, hospitality, education, and access to some traditional welfare services. Old people who attend 'The Adelaide' have the status of club members (Isle of Wight 1985). And Islington is demonstrating the value of neighbourhood offices which provide various municipal services for all client groups – at the local level (London Borough of Islington 1986). Neighbourhood officers will undoubtedly find it necessary to make the best use of all service possibilities, including the local old people's home, as clients start to place increased demands upon them. The style and history of this decentralization exercise proclaims the importance of client choice and control. It is inevitable that this will start to influence the character and lifestyle in the local residential home. Thus the possibility of including old age homes in a programme of radical reform becomes practicable.

The interesting and important point to be made about these initiatives is that, like the residential home, they display an ideal, or a set of ideals, which are translated in practical terms as a 'bricks and mortar' solution. However, having drawn such a comparison between residential settings and these facilities, there is an important difference. These three examples of innovations appear to be successful in that they are popular with and well-used by their local communities. It could be argued that in these instances the philosophy upon which the particular service provision is founded is relatively well 'embedded' in the physical structure of the facility. This is not simply a result of good design at the physical level – not everyone would agree that all features in all these buildings embody 'good design'. Nevertheless, it would seem that a level of integration of philosophy, function, and design has been achieved which leads to an acceptance by the client groups. We might go further to suggest that this springs from an understanding by the client of the philosophy which underpins the service itself, and the function that the building is intended to fulfil. In contrast, we have argued in this book that the residential setting does not enjoy this kind of endorsement from its 'constituents' and that, despite the high standard to which many of the hundred buildings in the study were constructed, residential homes have not been adopted by or incorporated into their local communities.

It is likely that, despite capital constraints, additional residential homes will be designed and built in the future. In the light of our findings about residential settings, and if our arguments are valid that these new initiatives come to be tested, changed, and endorsed by community usage, we have grounds to hope that future residential buildings will express philosophies which users both understand and endorse. It is true, however, that the three initiatives we have cited serve populations which include those who are likely to be less vulnerable than the residential elderly. Nonetheless we should not assume that frail elderly people are unable to contribute to shaping the philosophies and physical structures which embody residential care.

Conclusion

The hidden agenda for any text on twentieth-century residential care must be to question its function and to challenge the continuing isolation and separation of institutions from the community and from normal patterns of everyday life — both in ideological and material terms. It has been argued here that the current status of community care and the high esteem it enjoys are to some extent predicated upon the deterrent ethos associated with traditional forms of institutional care. Yet the case against residential care remains 'unproven' insofar as much of our evidence for attacking institutions is based on their historical failure and present inadequacies. It does not deny the possibility of policy-makers constructing a better future, nor the capacity of a new generation of care professionals to create, imaginatively, a supportive environment where individual freedoms do not pose a major threat to the institution and where old people feel 'at home'.

The difficulty in evaluating the actual and potential contribution of residential care derives, in part, from a persistent failure to establish the nature of its role and purpose. Our analysis of social history tells us that the nineteenth-century model for residential care prescribed an institutional form to stimulate the work ethic and to punish the feckless. But, at the same time, changes in the family structure, social relations and living arrangements in the community were constructed around forms that would serve changing methods of production and the shift to urban living. It is only in contrast to the oppressive image of the

Victorian institution that we have allowed our sensitivities to be dulled to some of the more harsh and exploitative aspects prevailing in community settings.

Many old people experience deep fear and anxiety in their lives. With increased frailty they become uncertain about their ability to manage the daily round. The support from family and neighbours may become precarious as community life and the world of work are subject to change and increasing pressures. Once familiar neighbourhoods change their character and start to appear threatening. At the same time 'the lady from the welfare' – once an authoritative, friendly, and reliable professional visitor in the form of district nurse or social worker – now makes less frequent visits and tends to be displaced by a less qualified substitute. The growth of statutory support services in the community has been vastly outstripped by demographic changes and financial restraint to the point where care in the community becomes problematic.

Now, in the late twentieth century, the ways residential homes operate within a spectrum of care remain unspecified, other than as a default option which is designed to deal with residual problems of care. But we might speculate that the punitive elements of institutional care remain. In a similar way, a general increase in standards of living might serve to mask the hidden despair and material hardship that is generated by fragmented and uncaring social relationships in modern urban communities.

Is life on the streets of our inner cities the best fate to which we can expose this older generation? We could cite numerous examples of apparent failure in community life and this should create an obligation to challenge its use as a benchmark against which to measure institutional care. This in turn means that it is quite inappropriate to judge residential care adversely for not achieving levels of happiness that do not necessarily pertain outside the walls of the institution. It is important to develop independent standards, as is the case with *Home Life* (Avebury 1984) and to locate evaluative criteria with a clear view of an alternative society characterized by greater mutuality and caring amongst people of different generations.

It should not be any more difficult to construct such a way of life in an institutional setting than in the normal community. That is the task for positive and creative social work intervention. At a more pragmatic level it will not be possible, in the short term, to meet the range of need without recourse to existing institutional forms. In the long term a re-evaluation will be necessary in the light of shifts that have taken place within the spectrum of care. For the present, it is argued then, that something akin to the residential flatlet might provide one acceptable face of institutional security which can be enjoyed by those elderly people who choose it. And it is possible that such an alternative, with appropriate checks and regulation, could be achieved within the public or the private sector. A programme of change might require a series of movements in policy and practice along the following lines:

1 Innovation or adaptation of the physical form of homes to establish access to and control over personal territory for elderly people.
2 Changes in social arrangements and management within homes to define individual rights and acceptable risks; homes must respond in practical terms to the demands of 'normalization'.
3 An alternative management structure for social services departments to integrate service provision and service delivery for old people in the community and in the residential section – this must expose the arbitrary nature of the institutional boundary.
4 Revised training schemes for field and residential staff, both management and workers, to support this alternative form of institutional care as one option within the community care spectrum.
5 Changes in community influence on the running of homes and involvement in activities within the homes; this must be a major part of democratizing services and encouraging communities to win back the welfare institutions that historically they have subscribed to but never owned.
6 For the private sector, there must be appropriate use of monitoring and regulation procedures to allay public anxieties about standards, and to work towards equivalence of service.

In the absence of such a critical review and re-evaluation of the role and structure of residential care, our best endeavours to deal with haunting memories of the past are doomed to failure. Minor adjustments will not suffice to shift the balance of institutional control. If residential homes continue to serve as a substantial part of the care spectrum, then an improved residential response must be constructed: one that will acknowledge and compensate for the powerlessness of older people who are presently obliged to submit without question to society's caring solutions.

It is necessary to design those kinds of residential environments which assert the rights of old people to lead private lives in public places. This will capture the traditional essence of home which is then represented as but one more option within the spectrum of progressive community care. This in turn will provide the legitimation for building a form of social care which acknowledges the fundamental importance of responding to consumer choice, thereby respecting the rights and freedoms of individual elderly persons to achieve a happier old age.

The National Consumer Study in 100 Local Authority Old People's Homes

funded by DHSS (Works Division) (Ref. no.: JI/RI96/40/Dev 2.3)

The National Consumer Study was based on a representative stratified sample of 100 local authority residential homes in England in 1980. For sampling purposes data were collected with regard to 29 local authorities and the 1,000 homes in their catchment areas. The sample of 100 homes was selected from this population. The data sets produced during the course of this study are as follows:

DHSS statistics
Information from March 1978 RA2 returns was supplied by DHSS for the twenty-nine authorities chosen for study. These data were used to construct the sampling frame.

Local authority questionnaire
Additional sampling information was sought from the twenty-nine local authorities e.g. presence of group living in homes.

Homes postal questionnaire
A postal questionnaire sent out to heads of homes in the twenty-nine local authorities – approximately 1,000 homes. Questions focused on aspects of regime within the home. These data were also used at the sampling stage.

Data from the sample of 100 homes
Inspector checklist – a detailed site inspection collecting factual data on physical provision and design features. This checklist was based around the items covered by the 1973 Building Note.

Resident questionnaire
Structured interviews carried out with 1,000 elderly residents within the 100 homes. Resident populations in each home were stratified according to age and sex, and a proportionate stratified sample of ten residents was taken from each home. The resident questionnaire formed the basis of a user evaluation of existing architectural and accommodation aspects of residential homes. However, other data collected included resident health, well-being, attitudes to and experiences of home life, reasons for coming into care. An attempt was also made to identify any preferred design features in an 'ideal' old people's home. In order to reduce the length of interviews for elderly residents certain sections of the questionnaire were asked of only 500 residents.

Use of substitutes in resident interviews
Of the original sample of 1,000 residents, interviewers were unable to interview 308 residents. In just over half the cases substitution was attributed to resident's mental infirmity; in only 7 per cent of cases was there an actual refusal (see *Table*). A comparison between levels of mental and physical fitness in the original sample and actual sample indicates that respondents were somewhat more alert and less frail than average. A comparison of age and length of stay shows broad similarity between the original and actual sample.

Crichton Royal Behavioural Rating Scale (CRBRS)
The CRBRS was completed for the 1,000 residents interviewed within the 100 homes. The CRBRS consists of a series of items which measure levels of physical and mental frailty. The scale is completed by members of staff for individual residents.

Staff questionnaire – the staff questionnaire was designed to replicate topics covered by the resident questionnaire and to show how different aspects of home life would be experienced by senior and care staff. Interviews

Reason for not interviewing originally sampled resident

	frequency	adjusted percentage %
Refused	22	7.4
Ill at time of interview	46	15.4
Doesn't speak English	1	0.3
Too deaf – interview not started	37	12.4
Too deaf – interview abandoned	3	1.0
Mentally infirm – interview not started	142	47.8
Mentally infirm – interview abandoned	15	5.0
Dead	9	3.0
Blind	6	2.0
Speech difficulty	4	1.3
Resident not available	6	2.0
Left the home	2	0.7
Other	5	1.7
Not answered	10	–
Total	308	100.0

were carried out with 400 staff – 2 senior staff and 2 care staff from each home. Other areas covered included demographic characteristics, working life, social interaction in the home, staff well-being, environmental assessment by staff.

Regime – in order to check the accuracy of the regime assessment conducted through the home postal questionnaire, an independent measure of home environment was included in the staff questionnaire. This was completed by one member of the senior staff in each home.

Visual game – a visual technique using a series of picture cards to enable residents to make choices over aspects of the physical/social environments that they feel are important within an 'ideal' residential setting. For further details of this technique see Willcocks (1984).

The ranked visual game choices are outlined in *Table 15* on p. 136.

Interviewer checklist – a short schedule completed by interviewers to gain an impression of the atmosphere of the home environment from people who were 'casual visitors'.

Resident/staff listings
The original list of residents and staff drawn up for sampling purposes. The listings also contain items not covered by other documents, e.g. details of temporary residents, details of domestic staff, and ancillary workers. This information allows for the calculation of overall staff ratio in homes.

The detailed qualitative study
The extensive survey data were complemented by the detailed qualitative study undertaken in three homes chosen from the hundred homes. The basis for the selection of the three homes was the inclusion of a variety of features rather than a concentration of similar features. The detailed study included an observation study and a location study and was piloted in one home – not included in the original one hundred.

The observation study
The observation study focused upon life for the residents and staff *within* the home and its immediate site. The study included the observation of a full weekly cycle of events within the home with between 80 and 100 hours of observation. In addition the researcher focused on four particular aspects of home life:

1 Meal-times – including the kitchen arrangements and those for provisioning the home
2 Bath-time – including staff allocation and organization of time
3 The management of incontinence – including laundry facilities
4 The management of physical deterioration and death

The location study
The aim of the location study was to provide information concerning the *external* environment of the residential home giving an indication of the importance of location and site for both residents and staff, and the level of community integration. Methods included a mapping exercise, group discussions with residents and staff; interviews with key officials e.g. architects, planners, homes advisers, and a small community survey with a sample of neighbours.

The neighbourhood questionnaire
Undertaken with twenty neighbours living adjacent to or within sight of each of the four homes. The schedule covered aspects of community life – amenities, traffic flow, safety, and how the area had changed over time. It also considered the image conveyed by the home, community participation with the home, and feelings about residential care for the elderly.

Longitudinal data about residents
As information concerning residents in the three homes chosen for detailed study was obtained at three stages during the research (during sampling, at observation, and at the location study), the opportunity was taken to assess changes in the resident population which had taken place during a year. The rate of 'turnover' and occupancy was calculated and analysis of CRBRS assessments over time gave an insight into changing levels of dependency.

For further details of the methodology and frequency counts for all surveys see Willcocks, D.M., Ring, A.J., Kellaher, L.A., and Peace, S.M. (1982) *The Residential Life of Old People: A Study of 100 Local Authority Homes*, Vol. II Appendices, Research Report 13, Survey Research Unit, Polytechnic of North London.

APPENDIX 2

The National Consumer Study in 100 Local Authority Old People's Homes, Secondary Analysis

During the period September, 1983 to November, 1985 secondary analysis of data from the National Consumer Study in 100 Local Authority Old People's Homes was supported by the ESRC (Ref. G00232019) and through ILEA Research Fellowships.

The main objective of this further analysis was the development of a model of residential care for the elderly, which sought to demonstrate the way in which resident well-being or resident lifestyle may be influenced by a group of factors relating to physical environment, organizational/social environment and resident mix (that is both the individual and collective characteristics of residents).

Our attempt to develop such a model involved the manipulation of both quantitative and qualitative data within a multivariate analysis. At the outset a decision was made to create a home-based data file in order to facilitate compatibility of data. Data from the original study consist of separate files for physical environment, residents, staff, and so on. Thus data from these separate files were transformed and transferred across to the home-based file. Further details of the secondary analysis are available in the final report to ESRC entitled *A Model of Residential Care: Secondary Analysis of Data from 100 Old People's Homes* and submitted in February, 1986 (Ref: G00232019).

The main data sets concerning physical environment, residents, and staff were submitted to the ESRC Data Archive at the University of Essex in August, 1986, and a user's manual is available from the authors at CESSA, Dept of Applied Social Studies, Ladbroke House, Highbury Grove, London N5 2AD.

THE DEFINITION OF COMPLEX VARIABLES USED IN THE TEXT

Choice – Range 0–11

Source: Staff questionnaire; homes postal questionnaire.
Derivation: Additive score with 1 valid case per home.
Items included:

Do residents have somewhere to lock up their personal possessions? *Yes* = 1

Is there a fairly set time at which residents are awakened in the morning? *No* = 1

Is there a fairly set time at which residents are expected to go to bed at night? *No* = 1

Can residents have breakfast . . .   *Choose time every day?* = 2
Choose time some days? = 1

Are residents encouraged to use their bedrooms . . .
Whenever they want? = 1

Are residents encouraged to bring their own furniture? *Yes* = 1

Is there somewhere residents can make a cup of tea or coffee? *Yes* = 1

Is there a telephone available for residents' use? *Yes* = 1

Can residents come and go outside the home
Whenever they wish? = 1

Can visitors come only at set times, or   *At any time* = 1

Privacy – Range 0–5

Source: Staff questionnaire; homes postal questionnaire.
Derivation: Additive score with 1 valid case per home.
Items included:

Do residents have privacy whenever they want? *Yes* = 1
Do residents generally have privacy for entertaining their visitors?
Yes = 1
Is there somewhere residents can make phone calls in private
(apart from main office)? *Yes* = 1
Do residents always have the same person to assist them at bath-
time? *Same person* = 1
Can residents lock their own rooms? *Yes* = 1

Involvement – Range 0–5

Source: Staff questionnaire.
Derivation: Additive score with 1 valid case per home.
Items included:

Do residents have a say in the general organization of this home?
Yes = 1
Do residents set up their own activities? *Yes* = 1
Are residents involved in planning menus? *Yes* = 1
Is there a handbook available for new or prospective residents
telling them how the home is run? *Yes* = 1
Is there a residents' committee held . . . *At least once a month* = 1

Engagement – Range 0–7

Source: Staff questionnaire; homes postal questionnaire.
Derivation: Additive score with 1 valid case per home.
Items included:

Do residents get a lot of individual attention? *Yes* = 1
Do staff members sometimes do things for residents that they
could do themselves? *No* = 1
Are residents taught new skills? *Yes* = 1

Can residents get along without doing very much for themselves?
$$No = 1$$
Do a lot of residents just seem to be passing time here? $\quad No = 1$

Do staff encourage residents to help themselves a lot, a little, or not at all? $\qquad A\ lot = 1$

Are staff encouraged to sit and talk with residents, as part of their job? $\qquad A\ lot = 1$

Physical amenities – Range 0–19

Source: Inspector checklist.
Derivation: Additive score with 1 valid case per home.
Items included:

If supplementary heating in . . . $\qquad All\ lounges = 2$
$Some\ lounges = 1$

If there is a WC (for both men and women) within 10m of . . .
$All\ lounges = 2$
$Some\ lounges = 1$

If there is a WC (for both men and women) within 10m of . . .
$All\ dining\text{-}rooms = 2$
$Some\ dining\text{-}rooms = 1$

If one bath for fifteen residents or fewer $\qquad = 1$
If one WC for four residents or fewer $\qquad = 1$
If all WCs have doors $\qquad = 1$
If there is a separate sluice room $\qquad = 1$
If there is a laundry $\qquad = 1$
If there is an ironing/sewing room $\qquad = 1$
If there is access to . . . $\qquad Residents'\ phone = 2$
$Staff\ phone = 1$
If bedside lights are provided for . . . $\qquad All\ residents = 2$
$Some\ residents = 1$
If bedrooms have socket outlets in . . . $\qquad All\ rooms = 2$
$Some\ rooms = 1$
If resident room could be used as a bedsitting room $\qquad = 1$

Socio-recreational aids – range 0–8

Source: Inspector checklist.
Derivation: Additive score with 1 valid case per home.
Items included:

View of street/garden then street/sea (i.e. interesting location) from all lounges	= 1
If there is more than one television	= 1
If there is a recreation room for hobbies/handicrafts plus bar	= 1
If there is a quiet room	= 1
If there is a visitors' room	= 1
If there is a garden for residents to sit in	= 1
If it is easy for mobile residents to get into the garden unaided	= 1
If there are chairs in the main entrance hall	= 1

Prosthetic aids – Range 0–14

Source: Inspector checklist.
Derivation: Additive score with 1 valid case per home.
Items included:

If there are handrails in . . .	*All lounges*	= 2
	Some lounges	= 1
If there are handrails in . . .	*All dining-rooms*	= 2
	Some dining-rooms	= 1
If one or more WCs are adapted for use by residents in wheelchairs		= 1
If one or more WCs are raised on platforms to assist residents who have trouble using WCs of normal height or if portable seat available		= 1
If WCs have handrails or grips . . .	*In all WCs*	= 2
	In some WCs	= 1
If corridors appear light or are artificially lit		= 1
If there are *no* steps or ramps, etc. in the corridors		= 1
If handrails in the main corridor are	*Continuous*	= 2
	In sections	= 1
*If there is a lift in the home		= 1
*If the lift can accommodate a wheelchair		= 1

(*Note: If home is single storey score 1 for both of these items)

Orientational aids – Range 0–5

Source: Inspector checklist
Derivation: Additive score with 1 valid case per home.
Items included:

If there is a residents' noticeboard	= 1
If any rooms are identified by signs	= 1
If any routes are identified by signs	= 1
If any rooms are identified by colour coding	= 1
If any routes are identified by colour coding	= 1

Safety features – Range 0–14

Source: Inspector checklist
Derivation: Additive score with 1 valid case per home.
Items included:

If there are emergency unlocking arrangements in bathrooms and WCs		= 1
If there is a call system . . .	*In bathrooms only*	= 1
	In WCs only	= 1
	In both	= 2
If there is a night light in residents' bedrooms . . .	*In all*	= 2
	In some	= 1
If there is a call system in residents' bedrooms and		= 1
If it can be reached from residents' beds . . .	*In all rooms*	= 2
	In some rooms	= 1
If the corridors are lit at night		= 1
If there are fire doors along the corridors		= 1
If there are smoke/heat detectors in corridors		= 1
If there is emergency lighting		= 1
If the bedrooms contain fitted furniture . . .	*All rooms*	= 2
	Some rooms	= 1

Architectural choice – Range 0–20

Source: Inspector checklist.
Derivation: Additive score with 1 valid case per home.
Items included:

If windows can be opened by the residents in . . .	*All lounges*	= 2
	Some lounges	= 1
If there is a lounge with no TV		= 1
If windows can be opened by residents in . . .	*All dining-rooms*	= 2
	Some dining-rooms	= 1
If there is a mixture of large and small tables in the dining-room		= 1
If the home has two of the following – ambulift, medibath, ordinary bath with grips		= 1
If there is a separate shower room in the home		= 1
If there is/are shower(s) in the bathroom(s)		= 1
If there are separate WCs for men and women	*All or some*	= 1
If there is a residents' shop		= 1
If there is a residents' tea-making room		= 1
If there is a chiropody/hairdressing room		= 1
If more than 50 per cent of residents have single bedrooms		= 1
If residents can control the heating in their rooms		= 1
If residents can open the windows in their bedrooms		= 1
If bedrooms contain wash-hand basins	*In all rooms*	= 2
	In some rooms	= 1
If there are locks on bathrooms/WCs		= 1
If there is somewhere for residents to lock away personal possessions		= 1

Space availability – Range 0–3

Source: Inspector checklist.
Derivation: Additive score with 1 valid case per home.
Items included:

If sitting/dining space per resident equal to or greater than $5.4m^2$	= 1
If size of a single bedroom equal to or greater than $10m^2$	= 1

If size of a double bedroom equal to or greater than 15.5m^2 = 1

Staff facilities – Range 0–7

Source: Inspector checklist.
Derivation: Additive score with 1 valid case per home.
Items included:

If staff use their own WC and not the residents'	= 1
If there is an office	= 1
If there is a staff common room/locker room/cloakroom	= 1
If there is a medical/clinic/doctor's room	= 1
If there is a duty room	= 1
If there is a staff house on site	= 1
If there is a staff flat/maisonette on site	= 1

Adjustment to home life – Range 0–8

Source: Residents' questionnaire.
Derivation: Additive scores computed for each resident. Home
score = mean score for ten residents interviewed in each home.
Items included:

When you first come to the home did you find it easy or difficult
to . . .

1 Learn to live with other people	*Easy*	= 2
	Difficult	= 0
	DK	= 1
2 Make friends with other residents	*Easy*	= 2
	Difficult	= 0
	DK	= 1
3 Get to know staff	*Easy*	= 2
	Difficult	= 0
	DK	= 1
4 Find your way around the home	*Easy*	= 2
	Difficult	= 0
	DK	= 1

Adjustment to ageing – Range 0–14

Source: Residents' questionnaire.
Derivation: Additive score computed for each resident. Home score = mean score for ten residents interviewed in each home. Items included:

All your needs are taken care of	*True* = 2
	False = 0
	DK = 1
You feel miserable most of the time	*True* = 0
	False = 2
	DK = 1
You no longer do anything that is of real use to other people	*True* = 0
	False = 2
	DK = 1
You never felt better in your life	*True* = 2
	False = 0
	DK = 1
You no longer have anyone to talk to about personal things	*True* = 0
	False = 2
	DK = 1
You are just as happy now as when you were young	*True* = 2
	False = 0
	DK = 1
Although you have some friends in (name of home) you still feel lonely at times	*True* = 0
	False = 2
	DK = 1

Residents' worries – Range 0–8

Source: Residents' questionnaire
Derivation: Additive scores computed for each resident. Home score = mean score for ten residents interviewed in each home. Items included:

Now during the past few weeks have you been worried about any of the following . . .

1 Worried about not having enough money for extras	*Yes* =	1
	No =	0
2 Worried about your family	*Yes* =	1
	No =	0
3 Worried about people you have trouble with in the home	*Yes* =	1
	No =	0
4 Worried about your health	*Yes* =	1
	No =	0
5 Worried about having a fall	*Yes* =	1
	No =	0
6 Worried about the way the home is run	*Yes* =	1
	No =	0
7 Worried about the safety of your possessions in the home	*Yes* =	1
	No =	0
8 Worried about being safe if there was a fire	*Yes* =	1
	No =	0

Worried about aspects of home life

This variable is derived from a subset of worry. Factor analysis of the responses to the items above revealed that two factors exist. Thus this variable consists of items 3, 6, and 7 – aspects of home life.

Dissatisfaction since coming to home

Source: Residents' questionnaire.
Derivation: This variable is based on two questions concerning resident life satisfaction before and after admission to a residential home. High values indicate that there has been a drop in the level of life satisfaction since admission. Again, these values are based on the average for the ten residents interviewed in each home. The two questions were crosstabulated to form one variable.

How satisfied are you with your life as a whole these days? All things considered would you say you are . . .   *Very satisfied* = 4
Fairly satisfied = 3
Not very satisfied = 1

Not at all satisfied = 0

DK = 2

And before you came to live here how satisfied were you with your life as a whole. Would you say you were . . . *Very satisfied* = 4

Fairly satisfied = 3

Not very satisfied = 1

Not at all satisfied = 0

DK = 2

Satisfaction with staff – Range 0–14

Source: Residents' questionnaire

Derivation: Additive scores computed for each resident. Home
   score = mean score for ten residents interviewed in each home.

Items included:

Do you ever feel that

1 Staff don't spend enough time talking to you	*Yes* =	2
	No =	0
	DK =	1
2 Staff are always telling you what to do	*Yes* =	2
	No =	0
	DK =	1
3 There are not enough staff in the home	*Yes* =	2
	No =	0
	DK =	1
4 There are too many staff in the home	*Yes* =	2
	No =	0
	DK =	1
5 You do not get to know the staff	*Yes* =	2
	No =	0
	DK =	1
6 Staff are always changing	*Yes* =	2
	No =	0
	DK =	1
7 Staff spend too long with particular residents	*Yes* =	2
	No =	0
	DK =	1

Job satisfaction – Range 0–96

Source: Staff questionnaire.
Derivation: Additive scores computed for each staff member. Home score = mean score for four staff interviewed in each home.
Items included:

I would like you to tell me how satisfied or dissatisfied you feel
   with each of these features of your present job . . .
   1 The physical working conditions
   2 The freedom to choose your own method of working
   3 Your fellow workers
   4 The recognition you get for your work
   5 Your immediate superior
   6 The amount of responsibility you are given
   7 Your rate of pay
   8 The opportunity to use your ability
   9 Relations between bosses and workers in residential care
   10 Your chance of promotion
   11 The way the home is managed
   12 The attention paid to suggestions you make
   13 Your hours of work
   14 The amount of variety
   15 Your job security
   16 Now taking everything into consideration how do you feel
       about your job as a whole.

Scoring   *Extremely dissatisfied* = 0
Very dissatisfied = 1
Moderately dissatisfied = 2
Not sure = 3
Moderately satisfied = 4
Very satisfied = 5
Extremely satisfied = 6

Psychological well-being – Bradburn's Affect Balance Scale
Source: Staff questionnaire
Derivation: Mean Bradburn Affect Balance Scores for the four staff interviewed in each home.

During the past few weeks have you felt

1	Particularly excited or interested in something	*Yes*	= 2
		No	= 0
		DK	= 1
2	So restless that you couldn't sit long in a chair	*Yes*	= 0
		No	= 2
		DK	= 1
3	Proud because someone complimented you on something you had done.	*Yes*	= 2
		No	= 0
		DK	= 1
4	Very lonely or remote from other people	*Yes*	= 0
		No	= 2
		DK	= 1
5	Pleased about having accomplished something	*Yes*	= 2
		No	= 0
		DK	= 1
6	Bored	*Yes*	= 0
		No	= 2
		DK	= 1
7	On top of the world	*Yes*	= 2
		No	= 0
		DK	= 1
8	Depressed or unhappy	*Yes*	= 0
		No	= 2
		DK	= 1
9	That things were going your way	*Yes*	= 2
		No	= 0
		DK	= 1
10	Upset because someone criticized you	*Yes*	= 0
		No	= 2
		DK	= 1

Staff worries – Range 0–14

Source: Staff questionnaire.
Derivation: Additive scores computed for each staff member. Home score = mean score for four staff interviewed in each home.

During the past few weeks have you been worried about

1 Not having enough money for day-to-day living   *Yes* = 2
    No = 0
    DK = 1

2 Relations with people at work   *Yes* = 2
    No = 0
    DK = 1

3 Your health   *Yes* = 2
    No = 0
    DK = 1

4 Your family   *Yes* = 2
    No = 0
    DK = 1

5 How things are going at work   *Yes* = 2
    No = 0
    DK = 1

6 Getting old   *Yes* = 2
    No = 0
    DK = 1

7 Worried about other activities   *Yes* = 2
    No = 0
    DK = 1

Worry about work

This variable is derived from a subset of the staff worry item. Factor analysis of the responses to the items above revealed that two factors exist. The variable 'worry about work' includes items 2 and 5.

Resident-oriented policies – Range 0–17

Source: Inspector checklist, staff questionnaire.
Derivation: Additive score with 1 valid case per home.
Items included:

There are both smoking and smoke-free rooms   = 1
There are some separate and some mixed WCs   = 1
Staff use residents' WCs   = 1

There are emergency unlocking arrangements = 1
There is a notice board = 1
Night lights are used only when necessary = 1
Residents can change the layout of their room = 1
Residents can bring their own furniture = 1
There are facilities in residents' rooms for locking away possessions = 1
Residents can choose the décor of their bedroom = 1
The home has a residents' committee = 1
Commodes are used only when necessary = 1
Residents are taught new skills = 1
Residents can plan their own entertainments and events = 1
Residents can design their own menus = 1
Residents can get up when they wish = 1
Residents can go to bed when they wish = 1

Staff-oriented policies – Range 0–12

Source: Inspector checklist, staff questionnaire.
Derivation: Additive score with 1 valid case per home.
Items included:

Separate WC for the staff = 1
Night lights are always on = 1
Commodes are used automatically = 1
Residents have no say in the running of the home = 1
Residents are not taught any new skills = 1
Residents do not organize their own activities = 1
Residents do not organize their own entertainment = 1
The planning of menus does not involve the residents = 1
A home handbook is not produced = 1
Residents get up at a set time = 1
Residents go to bed at a set time = 1
There are day attenders = 1

Main parameters of measures of outcome (scores converted to base of 100)

	high	maximum score	range	$\bar{x}$	sd	$\bar{x}$ score
residents						
adjustment to home life	easy to adjust	100	37–100	77.7	12.4	78
adjustment to ageing	well-adjusted	100	35–77	58.0	8.6	58
worry	high worries	100	1–44	18.0	8.2	18
worried about aspects of home life	high worries	100	0–42	9.8	8.8	10
dissatisfaction since coming to home	more dissatisfied after move	100	15–67	47.6	8.1	48
satisfaction with staff	dissatisfied	100	0–49	19.5	9.9	20
staff						
job satisfaction	satisfied	100	55–92	75.0	7.9	75
psychological well being	high positive	± 5	0–4.25	2.3	1.1	73
worry	high worries	100	0–39	14.3	9.3	14
worry about work	high worries	100	0–75	13.7	17.6	14

References

Abrams, M. (1978) *Beyond Three-Score and Ten*. Mitcham, Surrey: Age Concern England Research Publication.

Allen, I. (1983) *Short-Stay Residential Care for the Elderly*. Report No. 616. London: Policy Studies Institute.

Appleyard, D. (1969) Why Buildings are Known: A Predictive Tool for Architects and Planners. *Environment and Behaviour* 1: 131–56.

Appleyard, D. (1970) Styles and Methods of Structuring a City. *Environment and Behaviour* 2: 100–18.

Apte, R.W. (1968) *Halfway Houses*. London: Bell.

Atkinson, A., Bond, J., and Gregson, B.A. (1985) The Dependency Characteristics of Older People in Long-Term Institutional Care. Paper presented at the Annual Conference of the British Society of Gerontology, University of Keele, September.

Audit Commission for Local Authorities in England and Wales (1985) *Managing Social Services for the Elderly More Effectively*. London: HMSO.

Avebury, K. (1984) *Home Life: A Code of Practice for Residential Care*. Report of a Working Party sponsored by DHSS and convened by the Centre for Policy on Ageing under the chairmanship of Kina, Lady Avebury. London: Centre for Policy on Ageing.

Barrett, A.N. (1976) User Requirements in Purpose-Built Local Authority Residential Homes for Old People – the Notion of Domesticity in Design. Ph.D. Thesis, University of Wales.

Barton, R. (1966) *Institutional Neurosis*. 2nd edn. Bristol: John Wright and Son.

BASW (1978) *Residential Care: Report of a Working Party of the Social Services Liaison Group*. London: BASW.

Bebbington, A. and Tong, M. (1983) Trends and Changes in Old People's Homes: Provision over 20 years. Background paper for Seminar on Residential Care for Elderly People organized by DHSS, 19 October, London.

Bennett, R. and Nahemow, L. (1965) Institutional Totality and Criteria of Social Adjustment in Residences for the Aged. *Journal of Social Issues* 21: 44–78.

Beveridge Report (1942) *Social Insurance and Allied Services (The Beveridge Report)*. London: HMSO.

193

Bland, R. and Bland, R.E. (1983) Recent Research in Old People's Homes: A Review of the Literature. *Research, Policy and Planning* 1(1): 16–24.

Blenkner, M. (1967) Environmental Change and the Ageing Individual. *The Gerontologist* 7(3): 101–05.

Blythe, R. (1979) *The View in Winter*. Harmondsworth: Penguin Books.

Booth, T. (1983) Residents' Views, Rights and Institutional Care. In M. Fisher (ed.) *Speaking of Clients*. Social Services Monograph: Research in Practice. University of Sheffield.

Booth, T. (1985) *Home Truths: Old People's Homes and the Outcome of Care*. Aldershot, Hants: Gower Publishing Co.

Booth, T., Barritt, A., Berry, S., Martin, D., and Melotte, C. (1983a) Dependency in Residential Homes for the Elderly. *Social Policy and Administration* 17(1): 46–63.

Booth, T. and Phillips, D., with Barritt, A., Berry, S., Martin, D., and Melotte, C. (1983b) A Follow-Up Study of Trends in Dependency in Local Authority Homes for the Elderly (1980–82). *Research, Policy and Planning* 1(2): 1–9.

Booth, T., Phillips, D., Barritt, A., Berry, S., Martin, D., and Melotte, C. (1983c) Patterns of Mortality in Homes for the Elderly. *Age and Ageing* 12: 240–44.

Bowling, A. and Bleatham, C. (1982) The Need for Nursing and Other Skilled Care in Local Authority Residential Homes for the Elderly. *Clearing House for Local Authority Social Services Research* 17(9): 1–65.

Bradburn, N.M. (1969) *The Structure of Psychological Well-Being*. Chicago, Ill: Aldine.

Bradburn, N.M. and Caplovitz, D. (1965) *Reports on Happiness: a Pilot Study of Behaviour Related to Mental Health*. Chicago, Ill: Aldine.

Campaign for Mentally Handicapped People (1981) *The Principle of Normalisation: A Foundation for Effective Services*. London: Campaign for Mentally Handicapped People.

Campbell, A., Converse, P., and Rogers, W. (1976) *The Quality of American Life: Perceptions, Evaluations, and Satisfactions*. New York: Russell Sage Foundation.

Canter, D. and Canter, S. (eds) (1979) *Designing for Therapeutic Environments: A Review of Research*. Chichester: John Wiley & Sons.

Central Statistical Office (1981) *Social Trends 12, 1982*. London: HMSO.

Charlesworth, A. and Wilkin, D. (1982) *Dependency among Old People in Geriatric Wards, Psychogeriatric Wards and Residential Homes 1977–81*. Research Report No. 6, University of Manchester: Departments of Psychiatry and Community Medicine.

Clough, R. (1981) *Old Age Homes*. London: George Allen & Unwin.

Darton, R. (1984) Trends 1970–81. In H. Laming, R. Darton, D. Wilkin, R. Bessell, A. Butler, M. Johnson, I. Allen, A. Parker, and S. Hatch *Residential Care for the Elderly: Present Problems and Future Issues*. Discussion Paper No. 8. London: Policy Studies Institute.

Davies, B. and Knapp, M. (1981) *Old People's Homes and the Production of Welfare*. London: Routledge & Kegan Paul.

DHSS (1981a) *Care in Action: A Handbook of Priorities for the Health and Personal Social Services in England*. London: HMSO.

DHSS (1981b) *Growing Older*. Cmnd 8173. London: HMSO.

DHSS (1983) *Elderly People in the Community: Their Service Needs. Research Contributions to the Development of Policy and Practice*. London: HMSO.

DHSS and Welsh Office (1962) Local Authority Building Note No. 2. *Residential Accommodation for Elderly People*. London: HMSO.

DHSS and Welsh Office (1973) Local Authority Building Note No. 2. *Residential Accommodation for Elderly People*. London: HMSO.

DHSS and Welsh Office (1978) *A Happier Old Age: A Discussion Document*. London: HMSO.

Downs, R.M. and Stea, D. (eds) (1973) *Image and Environment: Cognitive Mapping and Spatial Behaviour*. London: Edward Arnold.

Equal Opportunities Commission (1982) *Who Cares for the Carers? Opportunities for those Caring for the Elderly and Handicapped*. Manchester: Equal Opportunities Commission.

Evans, G., Hughes, B., and Wilkin, D. with Jolley, D. (1981) *The Management of Mental and Physical Impairment in Non-Specialist Residential Homes for the Elderly*. Research Report No. 4. University of Manchester: Dept of Psychiatry and Community Medicine.

Fengler, A., Kellaher, L.A., and Peace, S.M. (1985) *The Meaning of Home for Elderly Widowed Homeowners: Consequences for the Decision to Move or to Homeshare*. Working Paper. Centre for Environmental and Social Studies in Ageing, Polytechnic of North London.

Finch, J. (1984) Community Care: Developing Non-Sexist Alternatives. *Critical Social Policy* 9 (Spring): 6–18.

Finch, J. and Groves, D. (1980) Community Care and the Family: A Case for Equal Opportunities? *Journal of Social Policy* 9(4): 487–514.

Finch, J. and Groves, D. (eds) (1983) *A Labour of Love: Women, Work and Caring*. London: Routledge & Kegan Paul.

Godlove, C., Richard, L., and Rodwell, G. (1982) *Time For Action: An Observation Study of Elderly People in Four Different Care Environments*. Social Services Monographs: Research in Practice. University of Sheffield: Joint Unit for Social Services Research and Community Care.

Goffman, E. (1959) *Presentation of Self in Everyday Life*. New York: Doubleday.

Goffman, E. (1961) *Asylums*. New York: Doubleday Anchor Books.

Goldsmith, S. (1971) Appraisal (of an Old People's Home). *Architects' Journal* 29 September: 704–13.

Graham, H. (1983) Caring: A Labour of Love. In Finch, J. and Groves, D. (eds) *A Labour of Love: Women, Work and Caring*. London: Routledge & Kegan Paul: 13–30.

Hansard (1947) *Parliamentary Debates*. House of Commons Vol. 444, 24 November, cols 1,603–718. London: HMSO.

Hanson, J. (1972) *Residential Care Observed*. London: Age Concern and National Institute of Social Work.

Harris, D. (1977) Seven Models of Residential Care. *Social Work Today* 9(1): 19–20.

Harris, H. and Lipman, A. (1980) Social Symbolism and Space Usage in Daily Life. *The Sociological Review* 28(2): 425–28.

Harris, H., Lipman, A., and Slater, R. (1977) Architectural Design: The Spatial

Location and Interactions of Old People. *Journal of Gerontology* 23: 390–400.

Harvey, D. (1970) Social Processes and Spatial Form: An Analysis of the Conceptual Problems of Urban Planning. Paper presented to the Regional Science Association.

Health Advisory Service (1982) *The Rising Tide: Developing Services for Mental Illness in Old Age*. London: Health Advisory Service, November.

Hiatt, L. (1980) Disorientation is More than a State of Mind. *Nursing Homes*. July/August: 30–6.

Hitch, D. and Simpson, A. (1972) An Attempt to Assess a New Design in Residential Homes for the Elderly. *British Journal of Social Work* 2: 481–501.

Home Office/Scottish Home and Health Dept (1983) *Draft Guide to Fire Precautions in Existing Residential Care Premises*. London: Home Office.

Howell, S. (1983) The Meaning of Place in Old Age. In G. Rowles and R. Ohta (eds) *Ageing and Milieu: Environmental Perspectives on Growing Old*. New York: Academic Press.

Hughes, B. and Wilkin, D. (1980) *Residential Care of the Elderly: A Review of the Literature*. Research Report No. 2. University of Manchester: Departments of Psychiatry and Community Medicine.

Hunt, A. (1976) *The Elderly at Home*. OPCS. London: HMSO.

Imber, V. (1977) *A Classification of Staff in Homes for the Elderly*. Statistical and Research Report No. 18, DHSS. London: HMSO.

Isle of Wight County Council (1985) *The Adelaide Club Handbook*. Isle of Wight County Council and Medina Borough Council.

Ittelson, W.H., Proshansky, H.K., Rivlin, L.G., and Winkel, G.H. (1974) *An Introduction to Environmental Psychology*. New York: Holt, Rinehart & Winston.

Johnson, M., Challis, D., with collaboration from Power, M. and Wade, B. (1983) *The Realities and Potential of Community Care*. Research contributions to the development of policy and practice: essays based on the seminar 'Support for Elderly People Living in the Community' sponsored by DHSS and held at the University of East Anglia, September 1982: 93–117. London: HMSO.

Kahana, E. (1974). Matching Environments to the Needs of the Aged: A Conceptual Scheme. In J.F. Gubrium (ed.) *Late Life: Communities and Environmental Policy*. Springfield, Ill: Charles C. Thomas.

Kellaher, L.A., Peace, S.M., and Willcocks, D.M. (1985) *Living in Homes: A Consumer View of Old People's Homes*. Centre for Environmental and Social Studies in Ageing, Polytechnic of North London and British Association of Service to the Elderly.

King, R.D. and Raynes, N. (1968) An Operational Measure of Inmate Management in Residential Institutions. *Social Science and Medicine* 2: 41–53.

King, R.D., Raynes, N.V., and Tizard, J. (1971) *Patterns of Residential Care*. London: Routledge & Kegal Paul.

Kleemeier, R. (1959) Behaviour and the Organisation of the Bodily and External Environment. In J.E. Birren (ed.) *Handbook of Ageing and the Individual*. University of Chicago, Ill: Chicago Press.

Kleemeier, R. (1961) The Use and Meaning of Time in Special Settings. In R. Kleemeier (ed.) *Ageing and Leisure*. New York: Oxford University Press.

Knapp, M.R.J. (1977) The Design of Residential Homes for the Elderly: An Examination of Variations within Census Data. *Socio-Economic Planning Sciences* 11: 205–12.

Koncelik, J.A. (1976) *Designing the Open Nursing Home*. Stroudsberg, Pa: Dowden, Hutchinson & Ross.

Korte, S. (1966) Designing for Old People, the Role of Residential Homes. *The Architectural Journal* 19 October, 144: 987–91.

Lawrence, R.J. (1982) Domestic Space and Society: A Cross-Cultural Study. *Comparative Studies in Society and History* 24(1): 104–30.

Lawrence, S., Walker, A., and Willcocks, D.M. (1986) *She's Leaving Home: Local Authority Policy and Practice Concerning Admission into Residential Homes for Old People*. CESSA Research Report. Polytechnic of North London.

Lawton, M.P. (1970) Institutions for the Aged: Theory, Content, and Methods for Research. *The Gerontologist* 10(3): 305–12.

Lawton, M.P. (1972) Assessing the Competence of Older People. In D.P. Kent, R. Kastenbaum, and S. Sherwood (eds) *Research, Planning and Action for the Elderly*. New York: Behavioural Publications.

Lawton, M.P. (1975) The PGC Morale Scale: A Revision. *Journal of Gerontology* 30: 85–9.

Lawton, M.P. (1980) *Environment and Ageing*. Monterey, Calif: Brooks/Cole Publishing Co.

Lawton, M.P. (1983) Environment and Other Determinants of Well-Being in Older People. *The Gerontologist* 23(4): 349–57.

Lawton, M.P. and Nahemow, L. (1973) Ecology and the Ageing Process. In C. Eisdorfer and M.P. Lawton (eds) *The Psychology of Adult Development and Ageing*. Washington, DC: American Psychological Association.

Lemke, S. and Moos, R.H. (1980) Assessing the Institutional Policies of Sheltered Care Settings. *Journal of Gerontology* 35(1): 96–107.

Lemke, S., Moos, R.H., Mehren, B,. and Gauvain, M. (1979) *Multiphasic Environmental Assessment Procedure (MEAP). Handbook for Users*. Social Ecology Laboratory, Veterans Administration. Medical Center and Stanford University School of Medicine, Palo Alto, Calif.

Levin, E., Sinclair, I.A.C., and Gorbach, P. (1983) *The Supporters of Confused Elderly Persons at Home*. London: National Institute of Social Work.

Lewin, K. (1935) *A Dynamic Theory of Personality*. New York: McGraw-Hill.

Lieberman, M.A. (1961) Relationship of Mortality Rates to Entrance to a Home for the Aged. *Geriatrics* 16: 515–19.

Lieberman, M.A. (1974) Relocation Research and Social Policy. *The Gerontologist* 14(6): 494–501.

Lieberman, M.A., Brock, V., and Tobin, S.S. (1968) Psychological Effects of Institutionalisation. *Journal of Gerontology* 22: 343–53.

Lipman, A. (1967a) Old People's Homes: Siting and Neighbourhood Integration. *The Sociological Review* 15: 323–38.

Lipman, A. (1967b) Chairs as Territory. *New Society* 9: 564–66.

Lipman, A. (1968) A Socio-Architectural View of Life in Three Homes for Old People. *Gerontologia Clinica* 10: 88–101.

Lipman, A. and Slater, R. (1977a) Homes for Old People: Towards a Positive Environment. *The Gerontologist* 17(2): 146–56.

198 *Private lives in public places*

Lipman, A. and Slater, R. (1977b) Status and Spatial Appropriation in Eight Homes for Old People. *The Gerontologist* 17(3): 250–55.

London Borough of Islington (1986) *Going Local: Decentralization in Practice.* Islington: Town Clerk's Department.

MacDonald, R., Qureshi, H., and Walker, A. (1984) Sheffield Shows the Way. *Community Care* 18 October.

Means, R. and Smith, R. (1983) From Public Assistance Institutions to 'Sunshine Hotels': Changing State Perceptions about Residential Care for Elderly People, 1939–48. *Ageing and Society* 3(2): 157–81.

Miller, E.J. and Gwynne, G.V. (1972) *A Life Apart.* London: Tavistock Publications.

MIND (National Association for Mental Health) (1979) *Mental Health of Elderly People.* London: MIND Publications.

Ministry of Health (1939) *Twentieth Report of the Ministry of Health for 1938–39.* Cmnd 6089. London: HMSO.

Ministry of Health (1950) *Report of the Ministry of Health for the Year ended 31st March, 1949.* Cmnd 7910. London: HMSO.

Ministry of Health (1955) *Ministry of Health Circular 3/55.* London: HSMO.

Ministry of Health (1968) *Annual Report for the Year 1967.* Cmnd 3072. London: HMSO.

Moos, R.H. (1974) *Evaluating Treatment Environments: A Social Ecological Approach.* New York: Wiley.

Moos, R.H. (1980) Specialized Living Environments for Older People: A Conceptual Framework for Evaluation. *Journal of Social Issues* 36(2): 75–94.

Moos, R.H. and Igra, A. (1980) Determinants of the Social Environments of Sheltered Care Settings. *Journal of Health and Social Behaviour* 21: 88–98.

Moos, R.H. and Lemke, S. (1980) Assessing the Physical and Architectural Features of Sheltered Care Settings. *Journal of Gerontology* 35(4): 571–83.

Moos, R.H., Gauvain, M., Lemke, S., Max, W., and Mehren, B. (1979) Assessing the Social Environments of Sheltered Care Settings. *The Gerontologist* 19(1): 74–82.

Murray, H.A. (1938) *Explorations in Personality.* New York: Oxford University Press.

National Assistance Act (1948) London: HMSO.

Neugarten, B.L., Havighurst, R.J., and Tobin, S.S. (1961) The Measurement of Life Satisfaction. *Journal of Gerontology* 16: 134–43.

Norman, A. (1980) *Rights and Risks.* London: Centre for Policy on Ageing/National Corporation for the Care of Old People.

Norman, A. (1984) *Bricks and Mortals: Design and Lifestyle in Old People's Homes.* London: Centre for Policy on Ageing.

Norman, A. (1985) *Triple Jeopardy: Growing Old in a Second Homeland.* Policy Studies in Ageing No. 3. London: Centre for Policy on Ageing.

Nuffield Foundation (1947) *Old People: A Report of a Survey Committee on the Problems of Ageing and the Care of Old People.* London: Oxford University Press.

Oakley, A. (1976) *Housewife.* London: Penguin Books.

Office of Population and Census Surveys (1982) *General Household Survey, 1980.* London: HMSO.

Office of Population and Census Surveys/Registrar General, Scotland (1983)

Census 1981 Persons of Pensionable Age, Great Britain. London: HMSO.

Pastalan, L.A. (1970) Privacy as an Expression of Human Territoriality. In L.A. Pastalan and D.H. Carson (eds) *Spatial Behaviour of Older People.* University of Michigan, Mich.

Patterson, E.A. (1977) Care-work: The Social Organisation of Old People's Homes. Ph.D. Thesis, University of Aberdeen.

Peace, S.M. (1981) Small Group Living Within Old People's Homes. Paper presented to XIIth International Congress of Gerontology, Hamburg.

Peace, S.M. (1983) The Design of Residential Homes – A Historical Perspective. Background paper for Seminar on Residential Care for Elderly People organized by DHSS, 19 October, London.

Peace, S.M., Hall, J.F., and Hamblin, E.R. (1979) *The Quality of Life of the Elderly in Residential Care.* Research Report No. 1. Survey Research Unit, Polytechnic of North London.

Pincus, A. (1968a) The Definition and Measurement of the Institutional Environment in Institutions for the Aged and its Impact on Residents. *International Journal of Ageing and Human Development* 1: 117–26.

Pincus, A. (1968b) The Definition and Measurement of the Institutional Environment in Homes for the Aged. *The Gerontologist* 8(3): 207–10.

Pincus, A. and Wood, V. (1970) Methodological Issues in Measuring the Environment in Institutions for the Aged and its Impact on Residents. *International Journal of Ageing and Human Development* 1: 117–26.

Pinker, R. (1971) *Social Theory and Social Policy.* London: Heinemann Educational.

Power, M., Clough, R., Gibson, P., and Kelly, S. (1984) Evaluating Volunteer Support to Elderly People in Residential Homes. *Research, Policy and Planning* 2(2): 14–20.

Rapoport, A. (1977) *Human Aspects of Urban Form: Towards a Man–Environment Approach to Urban Form and Design.* Urban and Regional Planning Series: Vol. 15. London: Pergamon Press.

Rapoport, A. (1982) *The Meaning of the Built Environment: A Non-Verbal Communication Approach.* Beverley Hills, Calif., London: Sage.

Rapoport, A. and Kantor, R.E. (1967) Complexity and Ambiguity in Environmental Design. *Journal of American Institute of Planners* 23: 210–21.

Raynes, N.V., Pratt, M.W., and Roses, S. (1979) *Organisational Structure and the Care of the Mentally Retarded.* London: Croom Helm.

Rosow, I. (1967) *Social Integration of the Aged.* New York: Free Press.

Rowles, G. (1978) *Prisoners of Space? Exploring the Geographical Experience of Older People.* Boulder, Co: Westview Press.

Rowles, G. (1981) The Surveillance Zone as Meaningful Space for the Aged. *The Gerontologist* 21(3): 304–11.

Rowles, G. (1983) Place and Personal Identity in Old Age: Observations from Appalachia. *Journal of Environmental Psychology* 3: 299–313.

Rowlings, C. (1981) *Social Work with Elderly People.* London: George Allen & Unwin.

Shanas, E. (1979) Social Myth as Hypothesis: The Case of the Family Relations of Old People. *The Gerontologist* 19(1): 3–9.

Sinclair, I. (1971) *Hostels for Probationers.* Home Office Research Studies No.

200   *Private lives in public places*

6. London: HMSO.
Sinclair, I., Levin, E., Neill, J., and Williams, J. (1983) Part III – Who Applies and Why? Background paper for Seminar on Residential Care for Elderly People organized by DHSS, October, London.
Smith, R.G. and Lowther, C.P. (1976) Follow-Up Study of Two Hundred Admissions to a Residential Home. *Age and Ageing* 5: 176–80.
Srole, L., Langner, T.S., Michael, S.T., Opler, M.K., and Rennie, T.A. (1962) *Mental Health in the Metropolis: The Midtown Manhattan Study.* New York: McGraw Hill.
Stevenson, O. (1981) Caring and Dependency. In D. Hobman (ed.) *The Impact of Ageing.* London: Croom Helm.
Thomas, N., Gough, J., and Spencerly, H. (1979) *An Evaluation of the Group Unit Design for Old People's Homes.* London: DHSS.
Tinker, A. (1984) *The Elderly in Modern Society.* 2nd edn. London: Longman.
Tobin, S.S. and Lieberman, M.A. (1976) *Last Home for the Aged.* San Francisco, Calif: Jossey-Bass.
Townsend, J. and Kimbell, A. (1975) Caring Regimes in Elderly Persons' Homes. *Health and Social Services Journal.* 11 October: 2,286.
Townsend, P. (1962) *The Last Refuge.* London: Routledge & Kegan Paul.
Townsend, P. (1981) The Structured Dependency of the Elderly. *Ageing and Society* 1(1): 5–28.
Ungerson, C. (1983) Women and Caring: Skills, Tasks and Taboos. In Gamamikow, E., Morgan, D., Purvis, J., and Taylorson, D. (eds) *The Public and the Private.* London: Heinemann.
Vladeck, B.C. (1980) *Unloving Care: The Nursing Home Tragedy.* New York: Basic Books.
Vroom, V.H. (1964) *Work and Motivation.* London: Wiley.
Wade, B. and Finlayson, J. (1983) Drugs and the Elderly. *Nursing Mirror* 4 May: 17–21.
Wade, B., Sawyer, L., and Bell, J. (1982) *Different Care Provision for the Elderly Research Project.* Final Report. Dept of Social Administration, London School of Economics.
Wade, B., Sawyer, L., and Bell, J. (1983) *Dependency with Dignity.* Occasional Papers in Social Administration No. 68. London: Bedford Square Press.
Wade, B., Finlayson, J., Bell, J., Bowling, A., *et al.* (1983) Drug Use in Residential Settings. Background paper for Seminar on Residential Care for Elderly People organized by DHSS, 19 October, London.
Weaver, T., Willcocks, D., and Kellaher, L. (1985) *The Business of Care: A Study of Private Residential Homes for Old People.* Research Report No. 1. Centre for Environmental and Social Studies in Ageing. Polytechnic of North London.
Westin, A. (1967) *Privacy and Freedom.* New York: Atheneum.
Wheeler, R. (1982) Staying Put: A New Development in Policy? *Ageing and Society* 2(3): 299–329.
Wheeler, R. (1986) Housing and the Elderly. In C. Phillipson and A. Walker (eds) *Ageing and Social Policy.* Aldershot, Hants: Gower Publishing Co.
Wilkin, D. and Jolley, D. (1979) *Behavioural Problems among Old People in Geriatric Wards, Psychogeriatric Wards and Residential Homes 1976–78.* Research Report No. 1. University of South Manchester Psychogeriatric Unit.

Willcocks, D.M. (1984) Consumer Research in Old People's Homes. *Research, Policy and Planning* 2(1): 13–18.

Willcocks, D.M. (1986) Residential Care. In C. Phillipson and A. Walker (eds) *Ageing and Social Policy*. Aldershot, Hants: Gower Publishing Co.

Willcocks, D.M., Peace, S.M., and Kellaher, L.A., with Ring, A.J. (1982a) *The Residential Life of Old People: A Study of 100 Local Authority Homes*. Vol. I. Research Report No. 12. Survey Research Unit, Polytechnic of North London.

Willcocks, D.M., Ring, A.J., Kellaher, L.A., and Peace, S.M. (1982b) *The Residential Life of Old People: A Study of 100 Local Authority Homes*. Vol. II. Appendices. Research Report No. 13. Survey Research Unit, Polytechnic of North London.

Wilson, M. (1984) *The College of Health Guide to Homes for Elderly People*. London: College of Health.

Wing, J.K. and Brown, G.W. (1970) *Institutionalisation and Schizophrenia*. Cambridge: Cambridge University Press.

Wyvern Partnership (1979) *An Evaluation of the Group Unit Design for Old People's Homes*. Wyvern Partnership/Social Services Unit, University of Birmingham.

Name index

Subject index